General Practice

———————— THE FACTS ————————

John Fry CBE, MD, FRCS, FRCGP
Elected Member 1970–92, General Medical Council

With the compliments of

SK&F

RADCLIFFE MEDICAL PRESS
OXFORD

© 1992 Radcliffe Medical Press Ltd
15 Kings Meadow, Ferry Hinksey Road, Oxford OX2 0DP

Reprinted 1993

A catalogue record for this book is available from the British Library.

ISBN 1 870905 43 1

Typeset by Advance Typesetting Ltd, Oxfordshire
Printed and bound in Great Britain by
T.J. Press (Padstow) Ltd, Padstow, Cornwall.

Contents

Preface

The National Health Service (NHS), and general practice in particular, is in a state of revolution and change. Its new targets are to achieve a more *effective* system with better health and less disease, a more *efficient* system with better use of resources and a more *economic* one that is better value for money.

The White Paper *Working for Patients* and the 1990 Contract created confusion and depression among health workers because of uncertainty and fears for the future. Such low morale has resulted from a lack of reliable data and facts.

It is truly amazing that Europe's largest employer, the NHS, with over one million workers, and with an annual cost of over £30 billion, should have existed and survived with so little available and published information and so few data for analysis, audit and action.

Yet, paradoxically, there is a considerable amount of data available if one knows where to look for it and how to translate and present it as something useful and meaningful.

Here, I set out the facts on general practice in the NHS and comment on their implications.

What data?

Demographic, epidemiological, operational and clinical.

Where from?

Chiefly from the various publications of the government health and social security departments and from my own studies and observations over 40 years.

Who for and how?

The data is presented clearly and simply, without statistical complexities, for 'ordinary' doctors, nurses, pharmacists, planners, managers and politicians.

Why?

This publication is timely because we are in the midst of changes and need basic facts in order to make decisions.

My aims are not only to inform but to stimulate and question and make my readers pause, ponder, think and consider.

How many doctors and GPs do we really need? What do GPs and practice nurses do and how much do they do? What are the most common conditions and which ones occur rarely? How does the UK compare with other countries in costs and health indices? Are all prescriptions really necessary? Why are there such variations in prescribing and referral habits among GPs?

I recommend my readers to enquire into the above by studying their own work and practices and to begin to find their way through the annual HMSO publications of *Social Trends*, *Health and Personal Social Services Statistics*, *General Household Survey* and the *Compendium of Health Statistics of the Office of Health Economics*.

JOHN FRY
September, 1992

Acknowledgements

To the above mentioned publications of the Department of Health, Office of Health Economics and Occasional Papers and reports of the Royal College of General Practitioners.

1

What is general practice?

General practice, or primary health care, is an essential part of every health care system in the world.

No matter what the system — private enterprise, prepaid insurance, a nationalized health service, or even a non-system in a developing country — there has to be someone, somewhere to whom a sick or injured person can turn to in the first instance.

That first-contact health worker needs to be a trained professional providing primary medical and health care.

Primary care

Primary health care, therefore, has to be the keystone base in an integrated system. It has to be part of the national, social and economic structure and:

- available
- accessible
- affordable
- appreciated and understood (by profession and public alike).

Its priorities must be to:

- cure, relieve and comfort (disease)
- promote (health) and prevent (disease and disability)
- rehabilitate (to health and fitness).

Structure

Whatever the system, the structure of health care provision involves four essential levels of care and management to populations. (*see* Figure 1.1)

Figure 1.1: Levels of care, population and administration

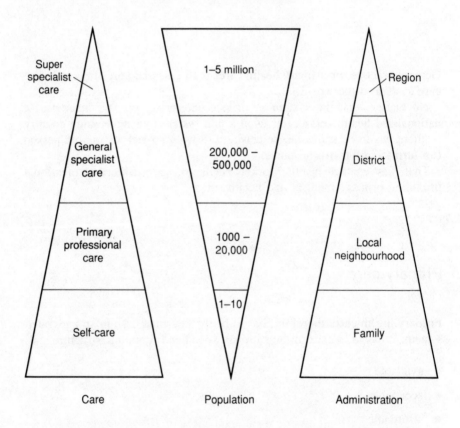

Care	Population	Administration

1 Self-care within a family of, say, 1–10 persons.

2 Primary professional care (or general practice) in neighbourhood localities for 1000–20 000 persons.

3 General specialist care by general specialists (ie surgeons, physicians, obstetricians, gynaecologists, paediatricians, trauma and orthopaedic

specialists, etc) in districts (based on district general hospitals) of 200 000–500 000 people.

4 Super-specialist care (ie cardiac, thoracic, neurological, etc) in regional units for populations of 1–5 million people.

Each level of care, including self-care, has its own:

- roles and functions
- content of morbidity and problems
- skills, tools, methods and techniques
- training, teaching and learning needs
- research, audit and checks on resources, quality and outcomes.

Features of British general practice

The characteristic features of British general practice are:

- single portal of entry into the NHS (except for accidents and emergencies and sexually transmitted diseases)
- direct access to 24 hour availability (for registered patients)
- first contact care involving diagnosis, assessment, triage and management or resolution of all defined problems
- co-ordination and manipulation of local medical and social services for individual patient and family needs
- gatekeeping and protection of hospitals through the selective referral system
- relatively small and stable population bases of 2000 patients per GP, or 10 000 per group of five GPs (on average)
- long-term and continuing generalist, personal and family care within the community, by doctors and health teams, of patients who come to know each other well over the years
- the content of clinical morbidity and mortality and of social problems and local needs will be those occurring in a population of 2000 or 10 000 (*see* Chapter 2)

● the GP has the opportunities to become the leader, provider and initiator
  of good health in his or her local community.

Flow of care

Taking all symptoms, illnesses and health problems in a community, three
out of four are self-managed by various means, with only one in four being
taken to the GP. Of the latter, only about one in 10 consultations lead to a
referral to the local hospital (*see* Figure 1.2)

Figure 1.2: Distribution of care

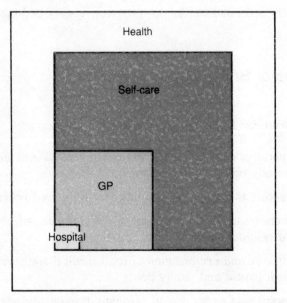

Figure 1.2: Flow of care

The flow of care in the NHS is through the single portal of direct access to
the GP and referral by him/her when necessary to hospital (*see* Figure 1.3).

Historical evolution of British general practice

The first references to a 'general medical practitioner' in social history
appeared about 200 years ago. Progress and recognition as a specialist field

Figure 1.3: Flow of care

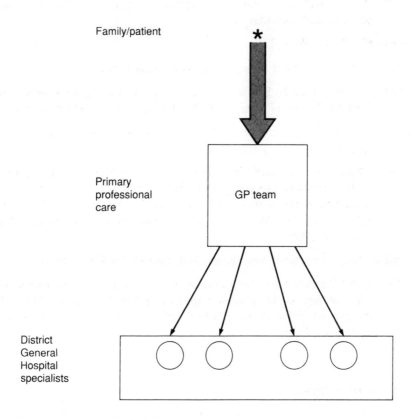

Family/patient

Primary
professional
care

GP team

District
General
Hospital
specialists

were slow and hard, largely because of intra-professional squabbles and jealousies. Some notable key dates are:

1815 Apothecaries Act recognized the Surgeon-Apothecary and the Society of Apothecaries (GPs)

1841 Royal Pharmaceutical Society of Great Britain (RPSGB) set up

1858 General Medical Council (GMC) set up to control standards, conduct and educate doctors and to protect the public and profession from quacks and lay healers

1911 David Lloyd George's National Health Insurance Act, providing compulsory prepaid health and medical insurance for employees below certain agreed low wages

1914–18 World War I

1920 Dawson Report setting out the future concept of health centres and primary and secondary care

1939–45 World War II

1942 Beveridge Report on setting up the Welfare State

1948 National Health Service set up under Labour government with Aneurin Bevan as Minister of Health (amidst reluctance from GPs)

1952 College of General Practitioners founded (amidst reluctance from specialists)

1966 Charter for General Practice, by government and profession, creating inducements with staff reimbursements, rent/rates reimbursements, seniority awards, higher rates of pay and items of service, pay for continuing education and for group practices (over three partners)

1982 Compulsory three year vocational training for GP principals

1990 New Contract for general practice with emphasis on better value for NHS money, audit, practice reports and leaflets, targets, attempted control of prescribing, hospital referrals, staff employment and budget holdings.

Practical issues

- General practice is the essential base level in all health systems, with its own roles, functions, features and tools.

- General practice within the NHS provides direct, available and accessible personal and family care to a small and stable community over many years.

- Historical evolution of general practice in the UK since 1815 has created a stable system of primary health care that is truly the envy of the world.

2

UK demography

Population

The population of the UK is 57.7 million and rising by about 0.15% annually, that is by 86 500 or 3 persons per GP per year.

Table 2.1: UK population by age

	under 5	5–14	15–29	30–44	45–64	65–74	75–84	85+	Total
Number of persons (millions)	4.0	7.3	12.7	12.1	12.7	5.1	3.1	0.9	57.7M
% of total population	7	12	22	21	22	9	5.5	1.5	100

Sources: Office of Health Economics and *Social Trends*

Table 2.2: Male/female ratios in the UK

Country	Male %	Female %	Total numbers (M)	Total %
England	23.6	24.6	48.2	83
Wales	1.3	1.5	2.8	5
Scotland	2.5	2.6	5.1	9
Northern Ireland	0.8	0.8	1.6	3
	28.2	29.5	57.7	100

Source: Office of Health Economics

Figure 2.1: UK population:age distribution

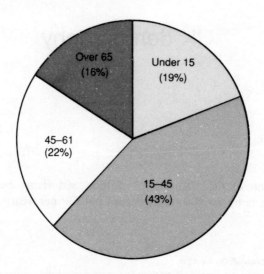

Figure 2.2: UK population by country and percentage

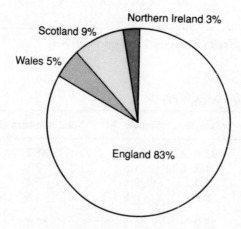

The proportion of over 65s in the UK is 16%, with variations between the four countries.

Table 2.3: Distribution of over 65-year-olds

Country	%
England	15.8
Wales	16.8
Scotland	15.0
Northern Ireland	12.5
UK	16.0

Source: Office of Health Economics

Life expectancy

The life expectancy (at birth) in the UK has almost doubled over the past 150 years. Babies born now can expect to live to over 70 years with males averaging 72.5 and females 78.8 years. in 1841 life expectancy was 40.2 and 42.2 years respectively.

Table 2.4: Trends in life expectancy 1841–1992

Year	1841	1901	1920	1943	1950	1970	1980	1990	1992 (estimate)
Male	40.2	48.5	55.6	61.6	66.5	68.8	70.4	72.2	72.5
Female	42.2	52.4	59.6	67.3	71.2	75.1	76.6	78.5	78.8

Source: Office of Health Economics

However, compared with other developed countries our life expectancy is only average.

Table 2.5: International life expectancies at birth, 1991

Country	Male	Female
Western European average	72.0	79.4
UK	72.5	78.8
USA	72.0	79.5
Australia	72.8	80.0
Canada	73.1	80.2
France	71.3	80.1
West Germany	71.1	78.7
Japan	74.9	80.3
Netherlands	73.3	80.3
Sweden	74.0	80.3

Source: *Social Trends*

Births

The birth rate in the UK has gone down almost three-fold in the past 120 years, but the infant death rate has been reduced almost 20-fold.

Table 2.6: Trends in birth and infant death rates 1870–1990

Year	1870	1900	1920	1940	1950	1960	1970	1980	1990
Live births per 1000 population	35.0	28.6	23.1	14.6	16.2	17.5	16.3	13.5	13.8
Infant deaths per 1000 live births	150	142.5	81.9	61.0	31.2	22.5	18.5	12.1	8.6

Source: Office of Health Economics

The total period fertility rate, ie total average births per woman in her reproductive years, has gone down and is now below the optimum of two required to keep the population stable at 57.7 million.

Table 2.7: Trends in family size 1951–91

Year	1951	1961	1971	1981	1991
Average births per woman	2.15	2.80	2.41	1.81	1.90

Source: Social Trends

Of all births, 25% are now to single (unmarried) women – until 1960 the rate was steady at 5%.

In 1987 there were 400 000 marriages in the UK and 165 000 divorces which suggests that one in three marriages ends in divorce.

Deaths

The crude death rate (includes all deaths) is 11.4 per 1000 population compared with 22.1 in 1870. In 1987 there were 651 000 deaths in the UK. The chief causes of death are:

- circulatory   49%
- cancer   25%
- respiratory   11%
- other   15%

Trends have been for circulatory and respiratory death rates to come down and cancer death rates to go up.

Practical issues

- Population of the UK is 57.7 million and rising by 0.15% a year due to immigration.

- 7% are children under 5, 16% are over 65 and 7% are over 75.

- 83% live in England, 5% in Wales, 9% in Scotland and 3% in Northern Ireland.

- UK inhabitants are living longer but not as long as in some other western countries. At birth boys can expect to live for 72 years and girls for 79 years.

- Birth rates are relatively low, as are infant death rates.

- On average women have less than the two babies required to maintain the population.

- One in three marriages is likely to end in divorce.

- One in four births is to an unmarried mother.

- Circulatory disorders account for 50% of all deaths, cancer for 25% and respiratory disorders for 10%.

3

The NHS

Historical

(*See* also Chapter 1)

To recap, the main historical events in the evolution of general practice and the NHS pre- and post-1948 (introduction of NHS) are:

Figure 3.1: Chronology of the NHS

```
                    ┌─────────────────────┐
                    │  1948: NHS set up    │
                    └─────────────────────┘
```

Pre-1948

- 1911 National Health Insurance Act (Local Insurance Committees)
- 1916 College of Nursing set up
- 1919 Ministry of Health set up Nurse regulations introduced
- 1920 Dawson Report (blueprint for health care)
- 1942 Beveridge Report – Welfare State
- 1946 Health Act (for NHS)

Post-1948

- 1950 Collings Report (critical of general practice)
- 1952 College of General Practitioners formed

- 1963 Gillie Report (health team)
- 1965/6 Charter for general practice
- 1974 Family Practitioner Committees (FPCs) set up (from Executive Councils)
- 1980 United Kingdom Central Council (UKCC) for nurses, midwives and health visitors formed
- 1982 Vocational training introduced for GPs
- 1985 FPCs become more independent
- 1990 New Contract
- 1991 NHS and Community Care Act

Levels of management

Management of the NHS can be related to levels of population (*see* Figure 3.2).

Figure 3.2: The NHS: managerial strata

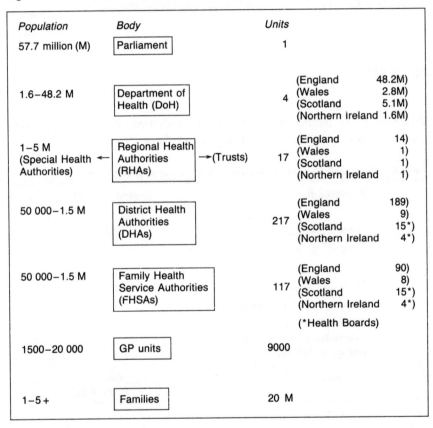

Population	Body	Units	
57.7 million (M)	Parliament	1	
1.6–48.2 M	Department of Health (DoH)	4	(England 48.2M) (Wales 2.8M) (Scotland 5.1M) (Northern Ireland 1.6M)
1–5 M (Special Health Authorities)	← Regional Health Authorities (RHAs) →(Trusts)	17	(England 14) (Wales 1) (Scotland 1) (Northern Ireland 1)
50 000–1.5 M	District Health Authorities (DHAs)	217	(England 189) (Wales 9) (Scotland 15*) (Northern Ireland 4*)
50 000–1.5 M	Family Health Service Authorities (FHSAs)	117	(England 90) (Wales 8) (Scotland 15*) (Northern Ireland 4*) (*Health Boards)
1500–20 000	GP units	9000	
1–5 +	Families	20 M	

(*see* also Figure 1.3)

Parliament is responsible for the whole of the NHS in the UK.

Department of Health (or equivalent). There is one each for England, Wales, Scotland and Northern Ireland, each with a Chief Medical Officer (or equivalent).

Regional Health Authorities. This is the management level between Departments of Health and the Districts.

District Health Authorities. These are responsible for district general hospitals and community health services.

FHSAs manage general practice and have more powers under the 1990 Contract.

General practices are independent and under contract to an FHSA.

Families take care of 75% of all health problems themselves.

NHS staff

The NHS is the largest civilian employer in Europe. It employs over one million people, or about one in every 40 workers.

Table 3.1: NHS staff (in percentages and overall numbers of employees)

Occupation	% (and units of 10 000 persons)
Nurses etc	50
Hospital doctors	6
GPs	3
Professional technicians	10
Managers and administrators	14
Domestic, works, maintenance, ambulance, transport staff etc	17
	100 (1 million)

Source: Office of Health Economics

Doctors

Doctors represent less than 10% of all NHS staff (3.3% are GPs and 5.5% are hospital doctors).

There are 33 000 GPs and 55 000 hospital doctors. Of the latter 20 000 are consultants and 35 000 are 'junior hospital doctors' (*see* Figure 3.3).

Figure 3.3: Doctors (types %)

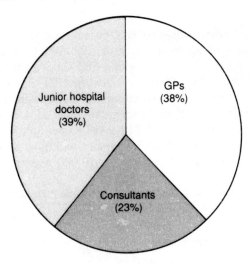

NHS hospitals

There has been a progressive reduction in the number of hospitals and in the number of available hospital beds (*see* Table 3.2).

Table 3.2: Number and capacity of NHS hospitals in 1959 and 1988

	1959	1988
Hospitals	3 000	2 050
Available beds	550 000	370 000

Source: Office of Health Economics

More than one in three of the population uses the NHS hospital service each year. The utilization rates per year are:

- admission to hospital, 13% of the population
- new referrals to a specialist out-patient department, 18% of the population
- attendance at an accident-emergency department, 23% of the population.

The practice team (*see also* Chapter 6)

There is no up-to-date published data, but estimates can be made. In 1991/2, with increased staffing as a result of the 1990 Contract, there are 2.5 employed staff per GP, or 1.7 whole-time equivalents (WTE) (the latter figure is still below the allowance of two per GP − *see also* Chapter 6).

In addition to these staff, district nurses, health visitors and midwives are attached to practices, and sometimes other specialist carers.

The whole team represents 3.7 (2.9 WTE) per GP, so that a partnership of five GPs will employ about 13 persons and have another six attached, making a team of some 20 persons for 10 000 patients.

Table 3.3: Primary care team: estimated numbers and WTE for UK (1991/2)

	Totals (persons)	WTE (whole-time equivalents)
GPs	33 000	33 000
Employed by GPs		
Managers	5 000	4 000
Practice nurses	18 000	10 000
Secretarial staff − receptionists and computer staff etc	60 000	42 000
Total	83 000	56 000
Per GP	2.5	1.7
Attached		
District nurses	21 500	21 500
Health visitors	14 500	14 500
Midwives	5 000	5 000
Total	41 000	41 000
ALL STAFF	123 000	97 000
Per GP	3.7	2.9

Costs

The total cost of health care in the UK must include NHS expenditure plus that spent on private health insurance and individuals' expenditure on medicines, health products, dressings etc.

Expressed as a proportion of the gross national product (GNP) total health care expenditure in 1990/1 was:

- NHS   5.85%
- Private   1.02%
  Total   6.87% GNP

Expressed in pounds sterling, the expenditure in Table 3.4 includes the amount spent per head of population. From this table it is evident that the NHS costs £520 per person per year, and another £30 per person is spent on private insurance (but only 10% of the population take up such insurance) and £61 on over-the-counter (OTC) pharmaceuticals and related products.

Table 3.4: Cost of health care in the UK, 1990/1

1990/1	NHS	Private insurance	Pharmaceuticals etc	Total
Cost (£)	£30 billion (B)	£1.75 B	£3.5 B	£35.25 B
Per head	£520	£30	£61	£611
% of total cost of health care	85%	5%	10%	100%

Sources: Office of Health Economics, Department of Health

Where does the money go?

Hospital services take up more than 50% of NHS expenditure (*see* Table 3.5) whilst general practice and its prescribing account for 20%.

The general practice total includes staff, premises and reimbursements, as well as GPs' income. If these divisions are disregarded, then GPs' prescribing costs are twice their net income — these proportions have existed since 1948.

The annual cost per head for the general practice service is £42 and for prescriptions £62. This means that each of the four consultations per year costs £10, plus £15 for medicines (the average per head of population).

International comparisons

Our health indices show that we have one of the cheapest and one of the most effective health care systems in the developed world.

Table 3.5: NHS expenditure (1990/1) by services in percentages and per capita

Service	% of total cost	Cost per head (£)
Hospitals	58	302
Community services	7	36
FHSA		
GP services	8	42
GP prescribing	12	62
Dental	4	21
Ophthalmic	1	5
Other	10	52
Total	100	520

Total cost of NHS = £30 B

Sources: Department of Health and Office of Health Economics

Table 3.6 shows the cost per head and the proportion of GNP spent by the major developed countries. In Japan and the UK, private expenditures were added.

Table 3.6: International expenditure per head and GNP % for selected countries (1987)

Country	£ per head	% GNP
USA	1252	11.1
Switzerland	1233	7.4
West Germany	1006	9.0
Sweden	1002	7.4
Canada	805	8.3
France	758	7.9
Netherlands	756	8.5
Japan	625 (+ private) =833	5.2 (+ private) =6.9
Italy	507	6.3
UK	423 (+ private) =486	5.8 (+ private) =6.87
World average per country	285	8.5

Source: Organization for Economic Co-operation & Development

Practical issues

- The NHS employs one million staff; doctors make up less than 10% and GPs only 3%.

- About 30% of the population use hospital services each year.

- Each GP has almost four health care staff; this means that a group of five GPs will have 20 co-workers.

- The NHS is not free — it costs £520 per head per year, plus another £91 per head spent on private medicines and private health insurance.

- However, the NHS is one of the cheapest health care systems in the developed world.

- More than 50% of the total expenditure is in hospitals; GPs and their prescriptions make up 20%.

4

What goes on in practice?

Content of work

Since general practice is the first level of primary professional care, its activities and content reflect the following (*see also* page 21):

● First contact care.

● Morbidity and mortality content of the small and stable population base.

Figure 4.1: Health care in a district of 200 000 persons

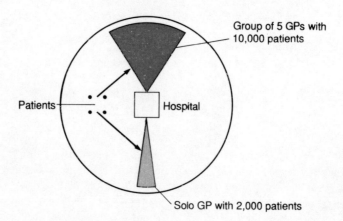

Thus, the average population base or denominator per NHS GP is 2000 persons and, since a typical group practice comprises four to five GPs, its population base is approximately 10 000. These are useful numbers to take into account when estimating numbers of likely clinical and preventive activities and social problems.

Spectrum of morbidity

In the NHS, general practice is the main entrance into the health care system so the content of morbidity is that which occurs in populations of 2000 and 10 000. The only selection will be for what patients decide to consult.

Some individuals and families carry out more self-care than others and consultation rates differ beween them.

The spectrum of disease and sickness in general practice is more representative than that in hospital practice because those attending hospitals are preselected for referral by GPs, except in the cases of accident-emergencies, sexually-transmitted diseases, and dental care.

Grade of illness

As most illnesses are minor, self-limiting and short-lived, there is a preponderance of such conditions in general practice; major life-threatening and disabling illnesses are less prevalent but more demanding of care. The middle group are of intermediate grade including many chronic disorders. (For the proportions of the three groups *see* Figure 4.2.)

Figure 4.2: Spectrum of morbidity

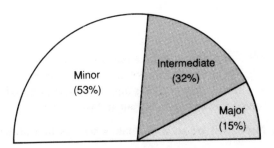

It should not be inferred from the high proportions of minor and intermediate grades that the GP is a 'mini-doctor'. Patients with these problems require as much skilled care and consideration as do those with more serious, major conditions.

What goes on in practice – 'a bird's eye view'

Taking the example population bases of 2000 per GP and 10 000 for a group practice, the likely content, pattern and demography of the practice will be as follows.

Population

There are more females (55%) than males (45%) in the population. The numbers of persons at various ages are as follows (*see* Table 4.1 and Figure 2.1).

Table 4.1: Age distribution of patients in the practice

Age	under 5	5–14	15–29	30–44	45–64	65–74	75–84	85+	Totals
per GP	140	240	440	420	440	180	110	30	2000
per practice	700	1200	2200	2100	2200	900	550	150	10 000
%	7	12	22	21	22	9	5.5	1.5	100

Annual birth rate

The present birth rate is almost 14 per 1000 so that in any year there will be:

- 28 births per 2000
- 140 births per 10 000.

Birth place

Although over 99% of births now take place in an NHS hospital most under supervision of the local specialist obstetric unit, almost all antenatal and postnatal care is 'shared' between GPs and specialists, and with the practice attached community midwife playing an important role.

Note: two in three will be to a woman who has had at least one child (a multipara).

Outcomes of pregnancy

Normal/natural delivery	80%
Assisted (forceps–vacuum) delivery	10%
Caesarean section	10%

For a GP with a list of 2000 patients there will also be:

- five legal terminations of pregnancy (TOP)
- five spontaneous abortions.

Thus, of all known conceptions:

- 74% will end with a child
- 13% will end with a TOP
- 13% will end with spontaneous abortion.

Figure 4.3: Outcome of conception

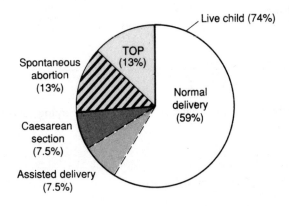

Infant mortality

This is now 8 per 1000 births. A GP with 2000 patients can expect such a death once every five years and a group practice with 10 000 patients one per year.

Annual death rate

The annual crude death rate is 11.5 per 1000, so that there will be:

- 23 deaths per GP with 2000 patients
- 115 deaths per group practice with 10 000 patients.

Where do people die?

In hospital	65%
At home	25%
In hospice	5%
Elsewhere	5%

Cause of death

Table 4.2: Causes of death

Annual deaths	per 2000	per 10 000
Heart disease	10	50
Cancer	5	25
Stroke	3	15
Respiratory disease	3	15
Others	2	10
Total	23	115

These numbers mean much care is needed for the dying, and also for the bereaved.

Clinical content of the consultation

The number of people who will consult in a year for the three grades of illness (minor, chronic and acute) are shown below for a GP with 2000 patients and for a group practice with 10 000. The sources are the National Morbidity Survey of 1981–2 and my own practice (Tables 4.3 to 4.8).

General minor

Table 4.3: Consulting rates for generalized minor conditions

Group	Persons consulting per year	
	per 2000	per 10 000
Upper respiratory infection	600	3000
Dermatological	300	1500
Rheumatic (musculo-skeletal)	230	1150
Minor trauma	210	1050
Psychiatric	200	1000
Gastrointestinal	150	750
Ophthalmic	90	450
'Symptoms'	320	1600

In all developed countries upper respiratory infections are the most prevalent cause of illness, but the high prevalence of dermatological, rheumatic and psychiatric conditions must also be recognized.

Specific minor

Table 4.4: Consulting rates for specific minor conditions

Condition	Persons consulting per year	
	per 2000	per 10 000
Acute throat infections	120	600
Backache	120	600
Eczema-dermatitis	100	500
Acute otitis media	92	460
Urinary tract infection	60	300
Ear wax	46	230
'Dyspepsia'	44	220
Migraine/headache	40	200
Hay fever	40	200
Vertigo/dizzy spells	30	150
Otitis externa	22	110
Constipation	18	90
Piles	16	80
Hernia (including hiatus hernia)	16	80

Note the high prevalence of backache, eczema-dermatitis, ear problems and urinary tract infections.

Chronic conditions

These 'chronic' or long-term disorders account numerically for much of the continuing care in general practice. Their numbers in a group practice are high enough to consider special clinics for those affected.

Gynaecological problems

These deserve a separate section as they are frequent and specific.

Table 4.5: Consulting rates for chronic conditions

Condition	Persons consulting per year	
	per 2000	per 10 000
Cardiovascular		
High blood pressure	100	500
Chronic IHD	40	200
Heart failure	24	120
Anaemia	14	70
(Pernicious anaemia)	(3)	(15)
Central nervous system		
Stroke (after effects)	20	100
Epilepsy	7	35
Parkinsonism	3	15
Multiple sclerosis	2	10
Cancers (under care)	15	75
Respiratory		
Asthma	36	180
Chronic bronchitis	22	110
Gastrointestinal		
Peptic ulcers	12	60
Irritable bowel syndrome	24	120
Diverticular disease	4	20
Endocrine		
Diabetes	20	100
Thyroid disorders	11	55
Chronic renal failure	1	5

Table 4.6: Consulting rates for gynaecological conditions

Condition	Number of women consulting per year	
	per 2000	per 10 000
Breast disorders	30	150
Vaginitis	40	200
Pelvic infections	5	25
Vaginal prolapse	10	50
PMT	20	100
Menopause	30	150
Menstrual problems	100	500
Sterility	6	30

Severe/major conditions

These are dramatic, acute and life-threatening.

Table 4.7: Consulting rates for major acute conditions

Condition	Persons consulting per year	
	per 2000	per 10 000
Acute bronchitis	116	580
Pneumonia	12	60
Acute myocardial infarction	8	40
(sudden death)	(4)	(20)
Acute stroke	6	30
Severe depression	10	50
(Parasuicide)	(4)	(20)
(Suicide)	(1 in 4 years)	(1)
Acute abdominal disorders	6	30
All new cancers	8	40

Cancers

Cancer is a frightening condition for patients and distressing for a doctor to diagnose. It is important to keep its incidence and outcome in perspective – eight new cancers per GP with 2000 patients per year.

Table 4.8: Diagnostic rates for cancers

New cancer sites	Patients diagnosed per year	
	per 2000	per 10 000
All cancers	8	40
Lung	1	5
Skin	1	5
Breast	1	5
Colon	2 in 3 years	3
Stomach	1 in 3 years	2
Rectum	1 in 3 years	2
Prostate	1 in 3 years	2
Bladder	1 in 3 years	2
Pancreas	1 in 5 years	1
Ovary	1 in 5 years	1
Lymphoma	1 in 5 years	1
Leukaemia	1 in 6 years	1
Cervix	1 in 7 years	1
Uterus	1 in 9 years	1 in 2 years
Oesophagus	1 in 10 years	1 in 2 years
Melanoma	1 in 10 years	1 in 2 years
Myeloma	1 in 12 years	1 in 2 years
Testes	1 in 15 years	1 in 3 years
Thyroid	1 in 25 years	1 in 5 years

Source: Cancer Research Campaign (1991)

The five year survival rate for all cancers is 40% and for specific sites as follows:

Table 4.9: Five year cancer survival rates

More than 50%		10–49%		Less than 10%
Skin	100%	Prostate	41%	Gall bladder
(Melanoma	60%)			
Breast	64%	Rectum	37%	Liver
Bladder	63%	Colon	34%	Lung
Cervix	57%	Leukaemia	23%	Oesophagus
Hodgkin's disease	53%			Pancreas
Uterus	52%			Stomach
Testes	51%			

Source: Cancer Research Campaign (1991)

Social pathology

In addition to clinical morbidity, social pathologies affect patients, their families and their doctors. It is important to appreciate their extent and their influence on patients' problems and difficulties.

Table 4.10: Social conditions of patients in the practice

Situation	Persons affected per year	
	per 2000	per 10 000
Poverty (grants)	300	1500
Unemployed	90	450
Homeless ('official')	5	25
One-parent families	30	150
Marriages	13	65
Divorces	5	25
Terminations of pregnancy	5	25
Alcohol + (more than 15 units/week)	15	75
Crime		
In prison	2	10
Juvenile delinquents	8	40
Burglaries	35	175
Drunken driving	5	25
Sexual assault	1	5

Source: *Social Trends*

Congenital conditions

In general practice there is concern to diagnose congenital childhood disorders as early as possible. However they are not frequent.

Effects of the 1990 Contract

The 1990 Contract has increased the GP's involvement with active prevention. Prevention used to take up 5% of the workload of general practice. This has now increased to about 25%.

Table 4.11: Diagnostic rates for congenital conditions

Condition	Diagnoses	
	per 2000 patients	per 10 000 patients
Squint	1 in 2 years	3
Undescended testis	1 in 5 years	1
Cardiac disorder	1 in 5 years	1
Mental retardation	1 in 7 years	1
Cystic fibrosis	1 in 10 years	1 in 2 years
Cleft palate	1 in 15 years	1 in 3 years
Spina bifida	1 in 15 years	1 in 3 years
CDH	1 in 20 years	1 in 4 years
Phenylketonuria	1 in 200 years	1 in 40 years

Table 4.12: Patients consulting for preventive reasons

Activities	Persons per year	
	per 2000	per 10 000
Childhood immunizations	150	750
Child surveillance	150	750
Cervical smear	120	600
Medical checks		
New registrants	150	750
3 year non-attenders	150	750
75+ elderly	130	650
Family planning	55	275

These are large numbers that may add an extra 10% or more to the numbers of attendances per year. A significant proportion take place during health promotion clinics.

Summary

- What is an ideal size of GP partnership for clinical, preventive and social work in general practice?

- Although over 50% of consultations in general practice are 'minor', the GP is not a 'mini doctor' – he/she is faced with chronic, acute-major and social pathologies.

- With 28 births per GP (with 2000 patients) and only five abnormalities (Caesarean section and assisted deliveries) the GP will have little experience of abnormal births.

- In addition to these 28 births, there will be five natural abortions and five legal terminations of pregnancy.

- Only one in four of all deaths (23 per GP with 2000 patients) now occurs at home and about 50% of these are acute and unexpected. Nevertheless, terminal care and bereavement counselling are important skills.

- The most prevalent clinical groups are upper respiratory infections, skin disorders, minor trauma, psychiatric and gastrointestinal disorders.

- Cardiovascular, respiratory and gastrointestinal disorders are the most prevalent chronic conditions.

- Acute chest infections, depression, myocardial infarctions and strokes are the most prevalent acute major conditions.

- Of the eight annual new cancers diagnosed by each GP, lung, skin, breast and colon make up more than 50% and the overall five year survival rate is 40%, but less then 10% for lung, stomach and pancreas cancers.

- The significant underlying social pathology must be seen as affecting the health of the community.

- The implications of preventive activities in the 1990 Contract are an increase in workload of more than 10%.

5

General practitioners

General practitioner principals form the largest group of senior doctors in the NHS − over 33 000 − compared with 20 000 consultants (*see* also Chapter 3 on the NHS).

GPs are now highly trained and highly paid. Each GP will cost the NHS over £2 million from the time he/she enters medical school until he/she dies on a pension in his/her mid-70s. The cost per GP will rise to over £10 million if fund-holding becomes the rule.

It is important therefore that we know how many GPs there are, who they are, where they are and, above all, how many we really need. At present it is not possible to answer this last question, but facts on the others can be examined.

Number of GPs

Table 5.1 gives the number of GPs in the NHS from 1950−92.

Table 5.1: GPs in the UK (1950–1992)

	1950(e)	1960	1970	1980	1985	1990(e)	1992(e)
GP principals	19 000	22 620	22 961	26 143	30 191	32 850	33 500
Assistants	2000	1335	727	305	266	250	300
Trainees	450	257	273	1704	1950	2000	1900
Total GPs	21 450	24 212	23 951	28 152	32 407	35 100	35 700
GPs per 100 000 population	43	46	43	52	57	62	63

(e = estimate)
Sources: Office of Health Economics [1989] and *Present State and Future Needs*, 6th ed [1983]

Comments

- The number of GPs per head of population has gone up by about 1.6 per year, meaning that the number of GPs has been increasing faster than the population.

- The number of GPs from 1970—90 went up by almost 2% per year.

- 1960—70 was a decade of crisis and demoralization for general practice with emigration and rejection of hospital specialties. The 1966 Charter changed this situation and entry into general practice has increased annually since 1970. In 1990—2 there was a decrease in the numbers of GP trainees as a result of the 1990 Contract (*see* Chapters 13 and 14).

- Assistantships were used as a form of training in the 1950s and 1960s but were replaced by organized vocational training (trainees) in the mid 1970s.

These ups and downs were also affected by the general morale and professional status and image of general practice. General practice has had a brighter image since the 1970s. It is now the first career choice of medical students and young doctors, partly because of the increasing restrictions on senior training posts for hospital specialties. In the 1970s and 1980s it offered good entry opportunities for many overseas doctors immigrating from Asia and Africa.

The population of the UK has been increasing by only 0.15% annually (it is 57.7 million in 1991—2) whereas the number of GPs has been increasing by almost 2% annually (*see* Chapter 2). This has meant smaller list sizes per GP (*see* page 34) with some knock-on effects on the volume of work per GP, especially because at the same time the practice team has increased in size (*see* Chapter 6).

At present there is some control on the number of new GPs entering practice through the Medical Practices Committee (*see* page 38) but the near 2% annual increase in numbers means around 500 new GPs per year.

List sizes

In the NHS patients register with a GP for care. Each GP is paid basically by capitation fees (ie per patient registered with him/her). There are also other contractual payments available. Therefore, it is important for GPs and managers to know the list size of each GP.

Table 5.2 shows the steady reduction of list sizes since the 1970s.

Table 5.2: Mean list size per NHS GP principal 1950–92

	1950	1960	1970	1980	1990(e)	1992(e)
Mean list size per NHS GP principal	2500	2257	2413	2189	1900	1875

(e = estimate)
Source: Office of Health Economics

The rate of fall (1.3% per year) has meant an average decrease of 30 patients per year on a GP list in the past 10 years, and if the rate continues, the UK list size will be around 1650 by 2001 AD.

There are national differences. Table 5.3 shows that since 1950 the average list sizes in England have been highest and in Scotland the lowest. Regionally too there are differences, but less so than in the past. There is now a much more even distribution of GPs. The highest list sizes in 1989 in England were in London in SW Thames (2065 patients per GP) and the NE Thames (2034) and in NW England (2051) and the lowest in Wessex (1885) and South Western region (1830).

Table 5.3: Mean list size per NHS GP principal for UK countries

	1950	1980	1985	1990(e)	1992(e)
England	2550	2247	2059	1960	1945
Wales	2450	2086	1914	1765	1750
Scotland	2220	1831	1688	1570	1555
Northern Ireland	1800	2097	1865	1760	1740
UK	2500	2189	2011	1900	1875

(e = estimate)
Source: Office of Health Economics

Another indication of the more even distribution of GPs is the class-ification of the Medical Practices Committee which is responsible for restricting the entry of new GPs into 'overdoctored' (restricted) areas.

However, it cannot direct GPs into 'underdoctored' (designated) areas. Table 5.4 shows that there are no underdoctored areas now and that almost 50% of GPs are in overdoctored areas.

Table 5.4: Distribution of general practices in England by list sizes (1968/1978/1988)

Classification of area	1968 %	1978 %	1988 %
Designated			
(average list size over 2500)	34	6	0
Open			
(average list size 2101–2500)	40	18	4
Intermediate			
(average list size 1701–2100)	16	36	52
Restricted			
(average list size less than 1700)	10	40	44
	100	100	100

Sources: Office of Health Economics and Department of Health statistical bulletins

Who are GPs?

Age

The average age of the general practitioner is going down. More young doctors are becoming principals and older doctors are retiring earlier (since 1990 the maximum retirement age for NHS GPs is 70 years). The proportion of GPs under 50 years old has risen from 58% in 1979 to 69% in 1989 (*see* Figure 5.1).

Sex

The number and proportion of women GPs is increasing rapidly. In 1950 the percentage of women in general practice was about 5%; in 1990 it was 25%, and by 2000 it is likely to be over 50%.

There are two reasons for these figures. Firstly, there are now equal numbers of male and female medical students. Secondly, more women doctors opt for general practice as first career choice (*see* Chapter 11).

Figure 5.1: NHS GP principals by age

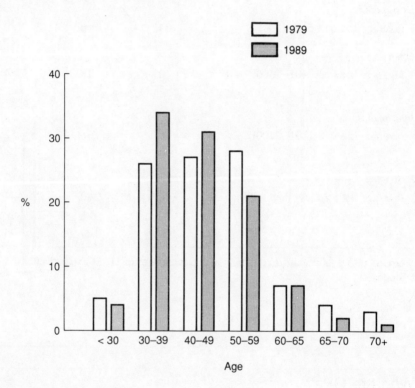

Place of birth

In the UK, 25% of GP principals (8000) were born and qualified overseas.

Table 5.5 shows that most 'overseas doctors' (ODs) are from the Indian sub-continent. Most came to the UK in the 1970s and 1980s and they represent a cohort now aged between 40 and 60. The 1990s may see an increase in numbers of GPs from EEC countries.

The highest proportions of OD principals are in NE Thames region (42% of all GPs) and NW England (32%), with fewest in SW England (6%) and Wessex (8%).

Figure 5.2: NHS GP principals: percentages of men and women

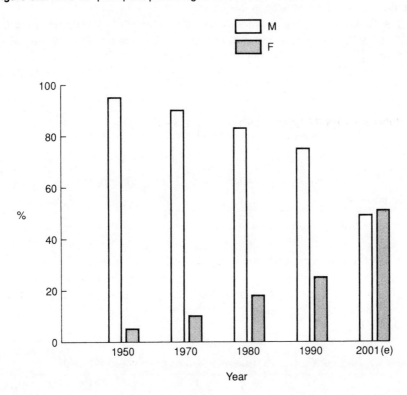

Table 5.5: NHS GP principals by place of birth

	1976 (%)	1989 (%)
UK	74.8	74.1
Irish Republic	6.5	2.8
Other − Europe	3.0	1.2
Indian sub-continent	11.4	16.3
Other − Commonwealth	2.3	3.4
Other	2.0	2.3

Source: Department of Health bulletins

Entry into practice – vocational training

In 1948 the NHS created the category of a 'GP trainee', who would be instructed as an apprentice by an approved trainer. However, the scheme was not popular because young doctors were permitted to practice as soon as they became registered.

The Charter of 1966 resulted in the creation of the vocational training (VT) programme, whereby trainees and trainers became better remunerated; and in 1982 it became mandatory for prospective GPs to go through the three year VT programme. As a result, the numbers of trainees and trainers increased.

Table 5.6: NHS GP trainees (index-linked) 1952–89
            (1952 = index of 100 with 309 trainees)

1952	1955	1960	1965	1970	1975	1980	1985	1989
100	98	85	40	68	234	551	623	618
(309 trainees)								(1908 trainees)

Source: Office of Health Economics

Table 5.6 shows the changes in numbers of trainees (using the year 1952 as the index take-off point) which illustrate the decline in popularity of general practice in the 1950s and 1960s, and the gradual influence of the 1966 Charter and impending mandatory VT in the late 1970s (*see also* Chapter 12).

Table 5.7: NHS GP trainers and trainees in England and Wales 1976–89

	1976	1978	1988	1989
Number of trainers	1441	1666	2778	2887
Number of trainees	819	1074	1877	1908
(UK)	(1225)	(1394)	(2228)	(2279)

Source: Department of Health bulletin

Table 5.7 shows the numbers of trainees and trainers (for the GP year of training only). In NHS history there have always been many more GP trainers than trainees (1.51 : 1 in 1989).

An additional reason for the increase in trainees is that general practice was the first career choice for 45% of pre-registration doctors in the 1980s (men 40% and women 53%) (Parkhouse, 1991).

Summary

GPs are the largest group of senior doctors in the NHS, and are an expensive commodity.

How many do we really need?

With more then 30 000 GP principals working for 40 years, from 30 to 70 years of age, the theoretical replacement requirement per year is less than 1000. However, many retire or die before they are 70. Therefore, a figure of 1500 is more reasonable. In fact, there are over 2000 GP trainees now being produced every year.

- **In relation to the population size and growth rate**, the numbers of GPs have exceeded population increases by a ratio of 1 : 1.6. In 1950 there were 43 GPs per 100 000 heads of population, and in 1992, 63 per 100 000.

- **Changes in numbers of GPs** are influenced by 'internal' NHS policies such as incentives, remuneration and conditions, and 'external' factors such as perceptions of status and image.

- **'Overseas doctors'** now make up over 20% of all GP principals – without them NHS general practice in the 1960s and 1970s would have been seriously undermanned.

- The proportion of **women GPs** is increasing and will continue to increase. In the 1950s about 5% of GPs were women, now 25% are women and by 2000 the figure may rise to 50%.

- **Average list sizes** have been decreasing since the 1960s. There are now 600 fewer patients per GP than in 1960. GPs in England have always had the largest lists in the UK, those in Scotland the smallest. The former each have 400 more patients on average than their colleagues in Scotland.

- There are no GP 'shortage areas' now and 50% of GPs now work in 'overdoctored' areas.

- Two-thirds of GPs are under 50 years old.

- Urgent planning is required to review numbers of GPs, particularly in view of the increase in roles for other members of the primary health-care team.

6

The health team

The evolution of the 'health team' has been a major part of British general practice in the NHS. The single-handed, do-it-yourself family doctor who worked from his home has been translated into a group practice; GPs supported by receptionists, secretaries, managers, computer operators, financial advisers, nurses, health visitors, midwives, psychologists and counsellors – plus cleaners, gardeners and maintenance persons – all working from a central building which may be a significant distance from some patients' homes.

These developments have been primarily prompted by the 1966 Charter. This laid out improved conditions for NHS GPs as a result of negotiations between the Labour government and the BMA. Group practices were to be encouraged financially, and staff salaries reimbursed by 70%. In addition, local health authority employed staff, such as district nurses, health visitors and community midwives, were to be attached to general practices. In some districts, associations would also be developed with local social workers and psychiatric community workers.

Who are the health team?

The general practice health team includes defined groups of workers, whose functions and roles need to be recognized and appreciated.

- **General practitioners** are the employers. They are in contract with their local FHSAs which reimburse 70% of the salaries of all the practice staff for whom employment has been approved. GPs are responsible by law for the acts of their employees.

- Many practices now employ a **manager** to run the business side of the practice and to organize the staff.

- With computerization, skilled **computer operators** are needed.

- **Receptionists** are the public face of the practice; they are patients' first point of contact. Receptionists receive calls, make appointments, give information and simple advice, relate closely with the doctors, and are responsible for record filing and distribution.

- **Secretaries** may double as receptionists or be involved exclusively in secretarial duties in communication and recording.

- The **practice nurse** has become a vital member of the team in the past five years and particularly since the 1990 Contract; the nurse's roles now include, in addition to traditional nursing, screening for early features of disease, health promotion, medical check-ups, cervical smears and immunizations.

- Some practices also employ dispensers, physiotherapists, psychologists, counsellors and others.

The 'attached' members of the team are employed by the local health authority:

- The **district nurse's** work is still mostly concerned with home visiting to the chronic and acute sick, but also with seeing patients on the practice premises.

- The **health visitor** still works with young mothers and their children in advising on and supporting better health.

- The **community midwife** is involved in the antenatal and postnatal care for all the maternity cases in the practice.

- In some districts, social workers, community psychiatric nurses (CPNs) and others may be attached.

From October 1993 health visitors and district nurses will have the right to prescribe.

How many members?

The size of the health team has doubled in the past 15 years. Proportionately the numbers of practice nurses have increased most markedly, now representing 12% of the health team members compared with 5% in 1976.

In 1976 the NHS stipulated up to two whole-time-equivalent (WTE) approved employees per GP. Although numbers have increased, the health team staff employed by GPs still amounts to 1.7 WTE per GP. However, FHSAs are now reluctant to allow more reimbursable staff to be employed because of the current financial situation.

The vast majority of receptionists and nurses in general practice are part timers, so that the acutal number of employed workers is 2.5 per GP or 1.7 whole-time equivalents, compared with 1.1 in 1976. The numbers of attached staff have increased, but these have only kept pace with increased numbers of GPs, so the WTE rate per GP has not increased since 1976.

The total health team of employed and attached members amounts to 3.7 (2.9 WTE) per GP, or around four to five actual workers (whole time and part time) per GP. This does not include special staff such as social workers, home helps, clinical psychologists and counsellors. Although not intimately involved with the GP team, these specialists often relate to the total care of the patient.

Pharmacists

Although not an integral part of the general practice health team, pharmacists are important primary care professionals who deal with more than seven NHS prescriptions per person per year (*see* Chapter 9). It has been shown that in developed countries (Kohn and White, 1976) at any time 33% of the population will be taking prescribed medicines, and another 33% taking over-the-counter self purchased medicines. Therefore, 66% of the population will be in contact with pharmacists.

Pharmacists' roles and potential in primary care have not in the past been fully developed or encouraged. They can and should play a more important part in collaboration with general practice, and a paper published in 1992 by the Royal Pharmaceutical Society of Great Britain (RPSGB) looked at ways in which this might be achieved.

There are over 12 000 'chemist and appliance contractors' in contract with FHSAs to supply NHS prescriptions (*see* Table 6.1). This means one for every 5000 persons, some being small while others form part of large stores.

It is against the law and against medical ethics for GPs to direct their patients to a particular pharmacy; nevertheless, it is likely that a practice will deal mainly with one or two local pharmacies. It would be sensible for a closer professional collaboration to exist between the two professional groups (medical and pharmaceutical) to develop joint general policies on health, disease prevention and management.

Table 6.1: Numbers of pharmacies and rates per population and GP

	1978	1989
UK total	11 489	12 363
per 100 000 population	20.4	21.7
per GP	0.4	0.4

Source: Health and Personal Social Services Statistics (1989)

A practice model

For a practice caring for a population of 10 000, the health team is likely to comprise:

GPs	5 (WTE)
	some may be part-time which would increase numbers

GP staff	
Receptionists	10 (part-time)
Secretaries	2
Managers	1
Practice nurses	3 (part-time)

Attached	
District nurses	3
Health visitors	2
Midwives	2 (part-time)

Others	2 (part-time)

Total	30

Comment

In 40 years general practice has progressed from a single-handed GP caring for about 2500 patients to a group model of five GPs, working together within a team of 30 providing services for about 10 000 people.

This has affected all the members of the team and the patients:

- Long-term personal and family care is more difficult for a team of 30 than in a single face-to-face relationship.

- Since personal care is the base of general practice, this should be a high priority for the practice.

- Management of the group, the premises, personnel, work and services, finances and patients have become more important and attention has to be paid to:

  who should lead?
  who should manage?
  who should make policy and detailed decisions?
  who should train and assess standards?
  who should check on outcomes and value for money?

Practical issues

- The past 40 years have seen the transition from single-handed practice to group practice with health teams.

- The health team includes members employed by the practice and whose salaries are variously reimbursed by the FHSA; attached nurses and others, employed by local health authorities; and associated groups such as social workers.

- Each of the above groups has its own recognizable roles, functions and skills which require regular checks and training.

- Practice nurses have almost quadrupled in number in the past 15 years. Their role has expanded and their contributions become more important. How much can and should they be asked to do?

- How should attached staff (district nurses, some practice nurses, health visitors and midwives) be integrated into the health team?

- How big should the health team be allowed to get? Should there be discussions on re-allocation of work? With nurses doing more work in the practice, how many nurses and how many doctors do we really need?

- There is one pharmacy to 5000 heads of the population and, with 66% of the population taking medicine daily, pharmacists are in close touch with individuals. Their role in primary health care should be greater.

- A typical general practice unit now consists of a team of about 30 members responsible for 10 000 registered patients.

- In the near future fundamental issues will need to be discussed relating to the 'health team':

  With such a large team of professionals, should GPs be the only partners? Should the 'team' become a 'partnership' with financial and business terms and implications?

  Should patients be involved and represented legally in the work and services of the primary care unit?

7

Practices

The organization and structure of practices has evolved from a 'cottage industry' to 'big business'. Merging of practices has led to fewer, centralized units — often much more than a 'pram-walk' distance for patients. Table 7.1 shows the trends since 1952 in partnership size.

The most remarkable change has been the reduction in solo (single-handed) practices. In 1952 almost 50% of all GPs worked alone; in 1989 the rate was one in 10 and falling. Likewise there has been a continuing increase in large practice units. In 1952 only one in 100 GPs was in a partnership of six or more; by 1990 the number was almost one in four and rising.

The changes have been influenced by the need for GPs to share facilities, including premises, staff and equipment, in order to provide better services and to make their own lives easier through rotas covering for out-of-hours work, holidays and non-practice duties, and the use of locum arrangements.

Table 7.1: NHS GPs in partnerships 1952–90

Partnership size (No. of GPs)	% of GPs					
	1952	1970	1975	1980	1985	1990(e)
1 (Solo)	43	21	17	14	12	11
2	33	25	21	18	16	15
3	15	26	25	24	21	18
4	6	16	18	20	19	18
5	2	7	10	12	15	17
6+	1	5	9	12	17	21
	100	100	100	100	100	100
Totals unrestricted NHS principals	17 204	23 697	25 191	26 907	29 663	32 250

(e = estimate)
Sources: Office of Health Economics and Department of Health statistical bulletin

Figure 7.1: Practice partnership sizes

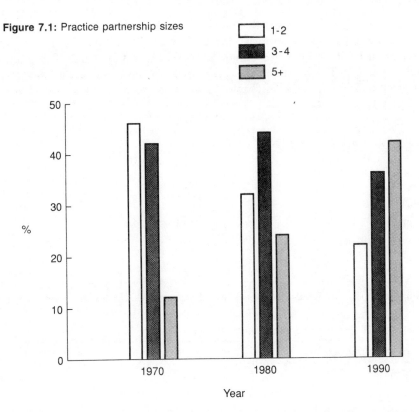

An added incentive for change was the 1966 Charter which introduced extra remuneration for GPs working in groups of three or more.

The mean partnership size of practices in 1952 was one to two GPs and in 1990 was four to five GPs. The number of practice units has consequently been reduced from almost 11 000 in 1980 to 9000 in 1990. Although only 10% of GPs are single-handed, they make up over 3000 GP units. A typical GP unit is now responsible for 8000–10 000 patients, whilst the largest practices have lists of over 20 000 patients.

Health centres

A major feature of the new NHS in 1948 was a blueprint for 'health centres'. These were to be purpose-built premises provided and managed by local authorities for rental by GPs. Although attractive in theory, they have not been popular with the majority of GPs, who have preferred to develop their own group practices and to own their buildings, often aided by attractive loans and support from the NHS through the cost-rent scheme.

However, Table 7.3 shows that one in three GPs now works from a health centre; there has been a slow and steady increase. The highest proportions of GPs in health centres are in Northern Ireland and Scotland. The mean number of GPs in a health centre is now over six, and there are a few very large ones with over 20 GPs. Table 7.2 gives the numbers of health centres in the UK.

Table 7.2: Health centres in the UK

	1980	1989
England	949	1233
Wales	84	93
Scotland	134	189
Northern Ireland	70	90
UK total	1237	1605

Sources: Office of Health Economics and Department of Health bulletins

Table 7.3: GPs working in health centres

% of all GP principals	1980	1989
England	23.7%	28.7%
Wales	30.5%	33.0%
Scotland	27.4%	38.9%
Northern Ireland	58.4%	58.5%
UK total	25.5%	30.1%
Number of GPs in health centres	6855	9777
Number of NHS GP principals	26 907	31 723

Source: Office of Health Economics

Practical issues

● With GPs choosing to be private independent contractors, the change from solo practice to group practice has been in their hands and has been relatively unplanned nationally or locally.

- The assumption has been that 'big is better'. Better for whom? Some **patients** have experienced a reduction in continuing personal care on a one to one basis. There is a danger that patients might be treated as 'cases' rather than people by the practice team.
  For **GPs** there are considerable advantages in better shared facilities and resources, with less stress through 24-hour cover and opportunities for regular professional contacts and surveillance.
  For the **NHS** it has been assumed that larger group practice is more cost-effective and of better quality, but there are no reliable data to support this.

- The growth in size of partnerships has been allowed with few controls and little guidance on what might be the **optimum size of a group**. One in four GPs works in groups of six or more partners, yet almost one in four still works alone or with just one partner. Much depends on local medical, social and health circumstances, but consensus guidelines should be produced.

- The number of **health centres** is growing. Their advantages and dis-advantages, compared with group practices, should be spelled out and future policies and plans discussed in each district.

- Closer collaboration with **local hospitals** should be developed by all practice units, including more shared care and records and use of the practice premises by hospital staff.

- Likewise the practice unit should take more responsibility for improving the health of its local **community** by collaborating with social and community services, and by encouraging patient participation.

8

The work

The content of general practice is presented in Chapter 4. Here I consider the hours and volume of work the GP and his team do, where it is done and by whom.

It is impossible to measure the extent of mental and physical stress to which GPs and their teams are subjected or its inevitable effects on performance.

It must be appreciated that general practice has evolved into team care and, although it is important to know the average GP's work rates, doctors are only part of the team, with nurses, receptionists and others sharing responsibility for caring for patients.

Measurements of 'quantity' are relatively easy; much more difficult are evaluations of 'quality' and 'outcomes' of work, bearing in mind that the overall *aim* must be health gain for the practice population.

The GP's volume of work

There are many components of general practice work. It includes consultations, home visits, answering the telephone, out-of-hours calls, administration, learning, teaching and discussion with others.

There follows an analysis of GP consultation and home visit rates. Relative proportions of each may be inferred from amounts of time involved (pages 53–6).

Uniquely under the NHS, people 'register' with a GP for care, enabling the population per GP to be known. It is possible therefore to determine numbers of consultations and home visits per individual and to compare the two figures.

It is also possible to calculate and produce a model of a typical day's work. Although the volume of work can differ greatly between individual practices, the majority fall within narrow medians.

Patient consulting rates

In any year 70% of all persons consult their GP at least once.
In any year 90% of families consult their GP at least once.
In five years the GP will treat more than 90% of his patients.

The **annual consultation rate per person** is the total number of consultations in the year divided by the GP's (or the practice's) registered
population (ie by the number of patients on his/her list). For example,
if there are 8000 consultations in a year in a practice of 2000, the annual
consultation rate will be 4.0.

GPs report a range of consultation rates between over six and under two.
The average consultation rates seem to be between three and four.

Fleming (1989) reported that in the National Morbidity Surveys the
rates were:

1955−6	3.7
1970−1	3.0
1980−1	3.5

The latest data, from the European study of referrals from primary to
secondary care, reports a rate of 3.3 for the UK. General Household
Surveys' extrapolations from periods of two weeks in 1989 set the rates at
four to five.

Regional reports in 1981 were:

Birmingham	3.2
Manchester	3.0
Merseyside	3.1

In my own practice, the annual consultation rates over 40 years were:

1950−9	3.5
1960−9	3.8
1970−9	3.2
1980−9	2.0
1990−2	2.5

Consultation rates by age

The young and the elderly consult most. In my own practice the annual consultation rates per person have been:

0–5	10–19	20–9	30–9	40–9	50–9	60–9	70–9	80+
5	2	2.25	2.5	3	3.5	4	6.5	8

Knowing the average annual consultation rate and the average size of the practice, it is possible to calculate approximate numbers of daily and weekly consultations.

Place

The proportion (and numbers) of GP home vists (house calls) has declined. In my practice, 95% of consultations now take place in the surgery, whereas in the 1950s 80% were in the surgery and 20% at the patients' homes.

Telephone consultations

These are not a feature of British general practice but in some countries of Western Europe, particularly Scandinavia, they may account for 20–30% of regular doctor–patient contacts.

Night visits

The image of the GP being called out nightly on home visits is, and always has been, a myth. Although the number of NHS night visit claims has increased, they are still at a rate of less than one per week per GP.

Night visits per GP per year

1967	1976	1989
(between 11 pm and 7 am)		(between 10 pm and 8 am)
11	24	38

(*Note*: extra 2 hours on-call in 1989)

It should also be noted that many GPs use deputizing services for their nightwork:

UK	45% of GPs
Manchester	90% of GPs
London	67% of GPs

Time distribution

Consultations and home visits account for two-thirds of individual items of a GP's work. Figure 8.1 shows the overall distribution of work-load.

Figure 8.1: Distribution of the work-load in general practice

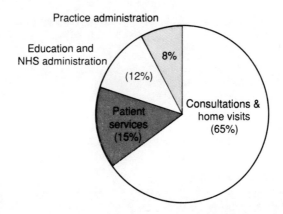

The Doctors and Dentists Pay Review Board has carried out two surveys (with 60% response rates) on doctors' time in practice, measured in hours spent each week:

Table 8.1: GP time on duty per week

	1985–6	1989–90
General medical service duties (GMS)	34.43	37.01
On call	27.46	23.48
Total	61.89	60.49
Other non-GMS	4.36	4.97

It has been noted that deputizing services carry out much on-call work for GPs; excluding these the work times per week were:

1985–6	38.79 hours
1989–90	41.98 hours

A further, more detailed breakdown of GMS duties showed the proportions of time spent on different types of work per week in 1989–90.

Figure 8.2: GP time distribution 1989–90

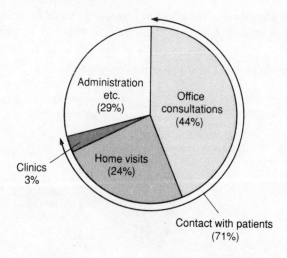

Table 8.2: GP time distribution per week

	% time
Office consultations	44
Home visits	24
Clinics	3
Teaching	1.4
Reading	4.2
Administration	6.7
Discussions over patients	14.1
Seeing pharmaceutical representatives	0.9
Other	1.7
	100
Total hours	37.01

Models

It is possible to produce models of consultation rates and time taken if the total numbers of consultations are recorded, and the practice population and average length of a consultation are known.

Table 8.3: Consultation rates for practice population of 2000

	Office	Home visits	Total
a) based on three consultations per person annually			
Per year	5100	900	6000
Per week	98	17	115
Per day	20	4	24
b) based on four consultations per person annually			
Per year	6800	1200	8000
Per week	131	23	154
Per day	26	4	30
c) based on five consultations per person annually			
Per year	8500	1500	10 000
Per week	163	29	192
Per day	33	6	39

It is also possible to calculate approximate amounts of time spent in consultations and home visits, based on the averages of 10 minutes per office consultation and 20 minutes per home visit.

Table 8.4: Time spent in consultation (hours) for practice population of 2000

	Office	Home visits	Total hours
a) based on three consultations per person annually			
Per week	16.5	6.5	23.0
Per day	3.3	1.3	4.6
b) based on four consultations per person annually			
Per week	22.0	8.5	30.5
Per day	4.4	1.7	6.1
c) based on five consultations per person annually			
Per week	27.2	9.7	36.9
Per day	5.5	2.0	7.5

Tables 8.3 and 8.4 show how GP time and work-load may be predicted, according to the practice's patient consulting rate, in order to optimize scheduling and planning for efficiency and patients' convenience.

The work of the practice nurse and manager

It is likely that practice and district nurses will undertake an increasing volume of work in the practice as a result of the 1990 Contract. They carry out:

- well person checks
- cervical smears
- immunizations
- health promotion clinics
- regular nursing tasks

Practice nurse profile

Mrs B is one of five part-time practice nurses in a large group practice, all of whom have different specialist fields. Her primary responsibilities are to run three clinics: for infant/child immunization, well woman screening and weight reduction.

Immunization clinics are run once a week for about 3½ hours, during which time up to 16 infants/children are immunized depending on attendance. All preparation and administration is carried out in this time. A doctor and health visitor are available for consultation if required.

Approximately 25% of the time is taken up with preparation, 25% with administration and 50% with immunization/consultation. The administration mainly consists of recording details of the immunizations, batch numbers of the vaccine and ensuring that the relevant records are copied to the patient's file and the child health computer at the local children's centre.

Well woman clinics take place once a week for about 3½ hours, during which time up to six patients are screened. Mrs B carries out urine analysis, measures blood pressure, records height and weight and gives advice on lifestyle and diet if required. She also instructs on breast self-examination techniques and establishes the patient's tetanus immunity, giving an immunization if necessary. The patients then have a cervical smear taken by a doctor.

Administration and preparation of each clinic takes approximately 40% of the time, with patient consultation (including smears) taking 60%. The administration mainly consists of recording patient details onto their notes and entering these observations and financial claims into the in-house computer.

Weight reduction courses take place three times per year for a duration of three months. The initial session runs for 4½ hours in which time up to 15 patients receive an initial consultation. Approximately 15% of the time is taken up with preparation and the remaining 85% is spent on consultations. Prior to the initial appointments, up to four hours are required to set up this clinic, which includes publicity, contacting patients and updating the waiting list.

In the subsequent sessions groups of up to 10 patients meet fortnightly for 1½ hours for weighing, discussion and counselling. Preparation and administration account for 15% of the time and 85% for the session itself.

All the above clinics follow the national trend of some unexplained non-attendance. A limited amount of over booking is one of the methods employed by the practice to assist in the cost-effective running of the clinics. Mrs B is investigating the causes of non-attendance and possible strategies to combat this waste of valuable resources.

As modern general practice becomes increasingly business-oriented, more partnerships are employing a professional manager. The roles of a practice manager in the primary care team can be as many and varied as there are general practices. However, the daily tasks of the **practice manager** should work towards the following objectives:

- To offer a high quality service to patients

- To encourage personal development for all members of the primary health care team

- To maintain a reasonable income for the practice.

The job involves:

- **Planning**. This should be long- as well as short-term and involve regular partnership meetings at which ideas may be discussed, policies thrashed out and decisions taken.

- **Managing people**. Communicating between GP partners, teambuilding for optimal efficiency and patient benefit, in-house training.

- **Patient services**. Co-ordination, evaluation (eg through patient question-naires), audit.

- Ensuring that services are **cost-effective**.

- Managing the **premises**.

- Developing suitable systems for **data collection and storage**.

Practical issues

- Amount of 'work' done is a highly sensitive topic. Whilst **quantity** by volume and numbers is relatively easy to measure, **quality** is much more difficult to assess.

- In the NHS it is possible to determine **patient-consulting** rates, ie proportions of population who consult in a year (70%), and **mean annual consultation rates**, ie total consultations divided by the regis-tered practice population. The mean rate is three to four, but with ranges of two to six. Why the extreme differences?

- The number and proportion of **home visits** has decreased considerably.

- **Night visits** (or claims for them) have increased; yet they amount to less than one per GP per week, and many are carried out by commercial deputizing services. Does this explain the increase?

- GPs' **working hours** are difficult to measure and apportion. It appears that face to face consultations with patients take up five to six hours per working day, and total work, including administration, teaching, learn-ing etc. adds up to less than 40 hours per week, plus time 'on call'.

- **Practice nurses and managers** have taken over many tasks which the GP used to undertake himself.

9

Prescribing

A least one prescription is given by a GP in two out of three consultations and numerous repeat prescriptions are given to unseen patients.

Prescribing of drugs by GPs is high in volume and costs. This is balanced by benefits in terms of prevention of hospital treatment, and the high costs this often entails, and by direct patient benefits. However, there is uncertainty over the real benefits of some medications prescribed.

It must be accepted that taking medicines is an extremely prevalent and popular human activity. In an international study it was found that at any time 66% of the world population are taking medicines — 50% of these are prescribed medicines and 50% bought 'over the counter' at pharmacies (Kohn and White, 1976).

The NHS pays for the bulk of prescriptions issued by GPs; certain bodies make co-payments. The following is the detailed data on their extent and content. It must be noted that prescriptions reported in Department of Health statistics refer to **items** prescribed and not to prescription forms issued by GPs which may contain many items.

How much prescribing?

The amount of prescribing has been increasing progressively in the UK over the past 40 years.

The numbers of prescriptions (items) **per person** are:

	1950	1960	1970	1980	1990
Annual prescriptions per person	4.8	4.7	5.5	6.6	7.7

As may be expected, many more prescriptions were given in 1990 to the over 65s (16.3 per year) than to young persons (4.6).

These rates of prescribing by GPs differed appreciably between the four countries of the UK, with Wales and Northern Ireland always higher than England and Scotland (*see* Figure 9.1).

Figure 9.1: Annual prescription rates by country in UK

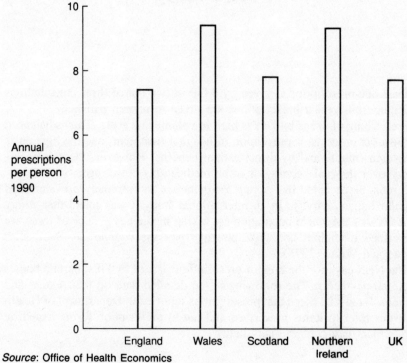

Annual prescriptions per person 1990

Source: Office of Health Economics

It is also possible to express the mean numbers of annual prescriptions issued **per GP**:

	1950	1960	1970	1980	1990
Total prescriptions per GP	10 955	9840	12 490	13 123	15 400

The rate for 1990 means that each GP writes out:

• 308 prescriptions per week

• 62 prescriptions per day.

Thus, each GP writes out twice as many prescriptions as the average number of patients that he sees in a day (50% during consultations and 50% for 'repeats' or for unseen patients).

What for?

The leading prescribed items, or groups of drugs prescribed, by GPs in 1978 and 1988 show how trends and habits change because of the introduction of new effective drugs and new policies.

Thus, the introduction of beta-blockers, calcium antagonists, ACE inhibitors, and other effective preparations for cardiac disorders, caused 'heart preparations' to go to the lead. Likewise the introduction of more effective anti-asthma drugs resulted in more prescribing for this condition. On the other hand, sedatives and tranquillizers, predominantly benzodiazepines, have decreased in use because of side-effects and risk of resulting litigation.

Figure 9.2: Leading prescribed items

	1978	1988
1	sedatives & tranquillizers	cardiovascular preparations
2	minor analgesics	dermatological preparations
3	dermatological preparations	anti-asthma drugs
4	penicillins	diuretics
5	diuretics	penicillins
6	cough medicines	minor analgesics
7	cardiovascular preparations	anti-inflammatory preparations
8	hypnotics	hypnotics
9	anti-inflammatory preparations	sedatives & tranquillizers
10	anti-asthma drugs	other anti-infective drugs

Costs

The GP drug bill has always accounted for about 10% of the NHS budget. In 1990–1 it will be over £3 billion. General practice prescribing makes up 82% of all prescription costs and hospital drugs 18%.

The cost of each prescription and the annual costs per person have escalated.

Table 9.1: Prescription costs in the UK, 1950–90

	1950	1960	1970	1980	1990 (e)
Cost per prescription (£)	0.17	0.37	0.68	2.99	6.50
Annual per capita cost for prescriptions (£)	0.81	1.74	3.76	19.90	50.50

(e = estimate)

Figure 9.3: The most costly and the cheapest groups of drugs in 1990

Average net ingredient cost per prescription for all groups:	**£5.77**
Drug group	*Cost (£)*
rheumatic	9.39
gastrointestinal	9.56
cardiovascular	7.12
respiratory	6.92
hormonal	6.84
analgesics (CNS)	3.00
ophthalmic	3.33
dermatological	3.35
for blood disorders (haematinics)	3.46
for infections (antibiotics)	3.98

International comparisons

Lest it be thought that annual costs of drugs per capita in the UK are exceptionally high, comparisons with other countries show otherwise.

Figure 9.4: International costs of drugs at manufacturers' prices (1987)

Country	Per capita annual cost (£)
Japan	172
West Germany	88
Switzerland	85
France	83
USA	75
Italy	72
Finland	62
Sweden	56
UK	**48**
Denmark	47
Netherlands	40
Norway	38
Spain	32
Greece	22

The numbers of items prescribed per head in the UK are also less than in other European countries.

Figure 9.5: International numbers of items prescribed (1989–90)

Country	Annual no. of prescribed items per capita (1989–90)
France	38.0
Italy	20.1
Portugal	17.1
Spain	14.8
West Germany	12.0
Belgium	9.3
UK	**7.6**
Denmark	6.1

Source: Association of the British Pharmaceutical Industry

Estimated prescription costs per GP (1990–1)

Figure 9.6: Annual prescription rates and costs in the UK

Number of prescriptions per patient	7.7
Cost per prescription	£6.50
Cost per patient	£50.50
Cost per GP of all prescriptions	£101 000*
Number of prescriptions per GP	154 000
*Note: gross income per GP was £55 485	

The total number of prescriptions per week per GP was 308, and the total per day per GP was 62. The cost of prescriptions written by a GP has been about twice his gross income since the start of the NHS.

Self-medication

Note: OTC = 'over the counter' prescribing.

What actions do people take when they develop problems and symptoms?

Figure 9.7: Responses to problems and symptoms

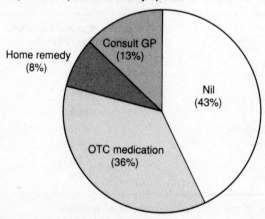

Source: Proprietary Association of Great Britain

At any time, on any day, 33% of the population are self-medicating and another 33% are taking prescribed medication.

The most frequent symptoms for which self-medication is undertaken are:

	%
tiredness	35
headache	30
aches and pains	25
overweight	20
backache	15
others	30

There is often more than one reason.

For **children**, the most frequent OTC preparations (in order) are:

- vitamins
- analgesics/antipyretics
- cough medicines
- skin applications
- laxatives

For **adults**, they are:

- analgesics
- vitamins
- cough medicines
- skin applications
- laxatives

Whilst GP prescribed drugs cost £3 billion in 1990, the amount spent on OTC preparations was £650 million.

Figure 9.8: OTC cost distribution

	%
Cough, cold, sore throat preparations	25
Analgesics	21
Vitamins	21
Indigestion, stomach upset, laxatives, anti-diarrhoeals	10
Skin applications	8
Other	15
	100
Total cost	£650 million

Summary

- In two of three consultations a prescription is written by the GP.

- The volume of prescribing has gone up. There are now 7.7 prescriptions per person per year − compared with 4.7 in 1960 − and at a cost of £6.50 per prescription, or £50.50 per person per year. The volume change has occurred because GPs are now treating conditions which used to be dealt with in hospital and are treating conditions which used to be untreatable.

- There have been changes over the years in levels of prescribing of different drugs. Sedatives and tranquillizers are now prescribed less and heart and asthma preparations prescribed more.

- Most expensive are prescriptions for rheumatic, gastrointestinal and cardiac drugs, and the cheapest are analgesics, skin and eye preparations.

- A GP writes on average 62 prescriptions per day, of which about 50% are for unseen patients or are repeats.

- Prescribing costs per GP − over £100 000 in 1990 − are twice the GP's gross annual NHS income.

- Per capita costs for drugs are less in the UK than in Japan, Germany, Switzerland, France, USA and Sweden.

10

GPs and hospitals

Health and medical care involves collaboration between GPs and hospitals, usually with the District General Hospital (DGH) and its general specialists.

Hospital utilization

Whilst only 5–10% of consultations involve referral to a hospital, the overall use of hospitals is much greater.

The number of hospital beds continues to fall despite the increase in utilization.

In 1989, 13.9% of persons were admitted to hospitals in the UK: 17.7% were newly referred to out-patient departments and 23.1% attended accident-emergency departments. There are no reliable national data on waiting times.

Table 10.1: Hospital utilization rates 1949–89

per 1000 population	1949	1959	1969	1979	1989
Hospital beds	10.3	10.6	9.5	8.0	6.5
In-patients	67	88	109	117	139
New out-patient referrals	140	159	166	167	177
Accident-emergency attendances	89	121	166	198	231

This means that in a practice of 2000 persons there will be per year:

patients consulting	1400
admitted to hospital	280
referred to out-patients department	360
attend accident-emergency departments	460

Figure 10.1: Hospital beds and patient attendances per 1000 population 1949–89

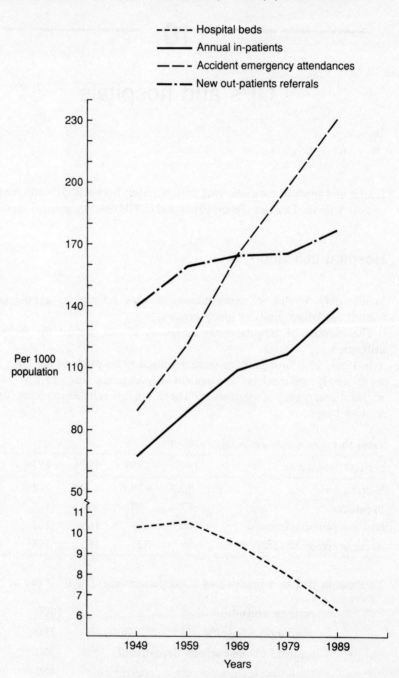

It is estimated that 33% of the population use hospitals at least once a year.

Domiciliary consultations

One of the facilities of the NHS is to allow the GP to call on consultants to carry out domiciliary (home) consultations on patients with problems that cannot be referred to out-patients departments.

In practice the *consultation* between GP and specialist originally planned for the NHS has become a *visit* by the specialist alone. The use of the *domiciliary consultation* scheme has been declining.

Table 10.2: Domiciliary consultations per year per consultant and per GP

Specialty	1978/9		1986/7	
	per specialist	per GP	per specialist	per GP
All	37	22	29	15
Medical				
Geriatric	217	–	187	–
General medical	78	–	52	–
Gastroenterology	63	–	35	–
Dermatology	63	–	49	–
Oncology	59	–	3	–
Chest	51	–	34	–
Rheumatology	49	–	42	–
Neurology	35	–	27	–
Paediatrics	25	–	16	–
Psychiatry	91	–	89	–
Pathology (haematology)	28	–	20	–
Radiology	15	–	14	–
Surgical				
General	54	–	36	–
Orthopaedics	45	–	30	–
Ophthalmology	23	–	15	–
Urology	20	–	11	–
ENT	19	–	9	–

Source: *British Medical Journal* (1988)

GPs *in* hospitals

There are two ways in which GPs are involved in hospital work:

- in community (GP) hospitals
- in District General Hospitals (DGH)

They operate as clinical assistants and hospital practitioners.

Community (GP) hospitals

There are 423 such hospitals in the NHS. They are distributed as follows:

England and Wales	350
Scotland	62
Northern Ireland	11

These provide care for 18% of the population and involve 16% of GPs who spend 10% of their time working in these hospitals.

GP appointments

In 1988 there were in the UK:

Hospital practitioners	950	(230 WTE)
Clinical assistants	8300	(2300 WTE)

Thus, the 9250 GP hospital workers represent 28% of all GPs.

Summary

- Although only 5−10% of consultations result in referral to hospital, in a year 14% of the practice population will be admitted one or more times: 18% are newly referred to out-patients departments, and 23% attend accident-emergency departments.

- Domiciliary consultations are declining, but still average 37 per year for a specialist and 22 for a GP.

- There are 423 community (GP) hospitals covering 18% of the population and involving 16% of all GPs.

- More than one in four GPs (9250) have clinical assistant or hospital practitioner appointments.

11

Women doctors

The NHS is the largest employer of women in the UK. Over 75% of its employees are women but they make up only 25% of principals in general practice. The proportion of women GPs is nevertheless increasing and within the next 20 years over 50% will be women. There are two reasons for this: 50% of all medical students now are women, and more women than men now enter general practice.

GP principals

In 1950 less than one in 10 GP principals was a woman; in 1990 24% were women.

Table 11.1: Percentages of women GP principals

	1950	1970	1980	1985	1986	1987	1988	1989	1990
% women GP principals	<10	10	17	19	20	21	22	23	24

Almost 50% of all trainees are now women. In 1990 46% of vocational trainees issued with certificates of satisfactory completion of training were women, out of a total of 2112.

Table 11.2: Women as percentage of successful GP trainees

	1981	1982	1983	1984	1985	1986	1987	1988	1989	1990
Women as % of trainees completing vocational training	39	38	32	35	34	38	40	40	42	46

Average list sizes

The average patient list sizes of women have always been smaller than those of men. In 1990 the average practice list size in England and Wales was 1962 patients. The average for men was 2119 and for women 1418.

Careers of women doctors

In a detailed and extensive study, Professor James Parkhouse reports on problems encountered by women GPs (Parkhouse, 1991).

He found that general practice was the first choice of new medical graduates of both sexes but that subsequent careers in practice were different for men and women.

10 years after graduating, out of those who entered general practice:

- 90% of *men* had become GP principals (96% with no break in their training)

- 61% of *women* had become GP principals (64% with no break in training)

It is of interest that more male than female GPs were married and had children.

Regarding employment status of women who had gone into general practice at the time of the survey:

- 40% were working full-time

- 47% were working part-time

- 8% were not working.

Of those with no children 83% were working full-time.

Parenthood had a marked effect on women's careers in general practice. 40% of childless women GPs had experienced a 'period of unemployment'; 63% of GPs with one or two children had been unemployed; and 77% of GPs with three or more children had been unemployed.

Problems

When questioned, women GPs reported many obvious problems interfering with their careers:

- having to give priority to their husbands' careers (often medical)
- pressures and stresses of domestic and family duties
- interruptions to and difficulties in attempting to carry out full-time post-graduate vocational training
- partners presenting problems regarding maternity leave.

It is clear that, since women doctors will soon be a majority in general practice, special consideration needs to be given to their career problems.

It is noteworthy that women vocational trainees do much better in the MRCGP examination than their male colleagues. The pass rate for women is 80% and for men it is 64%.

Practical issues

- It is likely that more than 50% of GP principals will be women in the foreseeable future.
- Attention must be given to the special problems that they encounter in their careers in general practice.
- Their training tends to be disrupted because of domestic and family duties, and difficulties created by their husbands' careers and the need for maternity leave.
- Part-time training and job-sharing in the practice have to be accepted as norms for the future.

12

Education and training

There are three stages in the education process:

- *undergraduate* – where medical students have a brief introduction to general practice

- *vocational training* for three years, which has been mandatory for NHS GP principals since 1982

- *continuing medical learning* which has always been one of the responsibilities of GPs.

Undergraduate

All the UK medical schools have implemented the recommendation of the General Medical Council that they should include some teaching on general practice in their curricula. All have departments of general practice; their courses differ. It is probable that the inclusion of such teaching has been partly responsible for motivating students towards a career in general practice.

Table 12.1 shows the number of students who have graduated from medical school each year since 1983.

Selection procedures vary between medical schools. It is evident that about one in 10 medical students do not complete their training and register within the five year allotted period. The cost of training and supporting (with maintenance allowances) a medical student is over £250 000.

Table 12.1: Students entering and graduating from medical schools 1983–90

	Entering	Register qualifications
1982–3	3994	3578
1983–4	3951	3498
1984–5	3996	3501
1985–6	3938	3483
1986–7	3967	3610
1987–8	3957	3595
1988–9	4015	3467
1989–90	4053	not available

Vocational training

The numbers of GP trainees have increased and have now stabilized in the UK at around 2000 a year. That means there are 6000 trainees at any time in the three year programme.

The three year vocational training scheme is under the supervision of the Joint Committee for Postgraduate Training in General Practice (JCPTGP), and this committee issues certificates of satisfactory completion of the prescribed course or for an equivalent programme.

The three year course includes two years in approved hospital appointments and one year in general practice under a recognized GP trainer.

Table 12.2: Trainer and trainee numbers in England and Wales

	1976	1979	1986	1989
Trainers	1441	1846	2769	2887
Trainees	819	1236	1814	1908
Ratio of trainers to trainees	1.76:1	1.49:1	1.53:1	1.51:1

The numbers of trainees and trainers have increased since 1982 when vocational training became mandatory; one practice in three is now a training practice and 12% of GPs are trainers (*see* Table 12.2).

JCPTGP

The Joint Committee has been issuing certificates since 1981. During the ensuing 10 years 21 553 certificates have been issued and 630 (3%) applications refused. Of those issued, 18 480 were for prescribed courses and 3073 for equivalents (to prescribed experience).

Table 12.3: Vocational training certificates issued 1981–90

	Prescribed (P)	Equivalent (E)	P:E	Male	Female	M:F	Total
1981	2376	186	93:7	1552	1010	61:39	2562
1982	2083	350	86:14	1512	921	62:38	2433
1983	1426	290	83:17	1171	545	68:32	1716
1984	1415	457	76:24	1221	651	65:35	1872
1985	1518	523	72:26	1341	700	66:34	2041
1986	1835	361	84:16	1354	842	62:38	2196
1987	2014	223	90:10	1341	896	60:40	2237
1988	1935	263	88:12	1319	879	60:40	2198
1989	1983	203	91:9	1256	930	58:42	2186
1990	1895	217	90:10	1147	965	54:46	2112
Totals	18 480	3073	86:14	13 214	8339	61:39	21 553

Source: JCPTGP report 1991

83% of successful students were from the UK, 13% from overseas and 4% from the EEC. Over 2000 certificates are issued each year, 46% of which were to women in 1990.

The most popular first hospital appointments were in obstetrics and gynaecology, accident and emergency, and paediatrics.

Royal College of General Practitioners

The total College membership in 1991 was 16 066, of which 1240 were fellows, 13 052 members and 1774 associates. 1052 were from overseas; 30% were women. This total represents just under 50% of all NHS GPs.

Membership of the College is by examination and in 1989–90 there were 1903 candidates with a pass rate of 74%.

Continuing medical education

In 1991 each GP was entitled under the 1990 Contract to spend up to £2000 each year on approved education. The Postgraduate Education Allowance (PGEA) would be reimbursable by the NHS. In 1991 over 30 000 principals therefore had access to over £60 million to buy education.

Summary

- All medical students now receive some education on general practice/ family medicine.

- General practice is the most popular career choice − preferred by over 2000 of the 4000 annual graduates.

- Vocational training for three years (one in general practice) is mandatory and there are over 6000 GP trainees at any time.

- At the end of approved vocational training, a certificate of satisfactory completion is issued by the JCPTGP. Over 2000 a year have been given over the past 20 years and 3% are rejected. In 1990 46% were given to women. 17% were given to doctors from overseas.

- Continuing postgraduate education through PGEA grants constitutes (potentially) a £60 million a year industry.

- With general practice the largest 'speciality' for over 50% of new medical graduates, continuing surveillance is necessary to ensure high standards of education and training, and value for money.

13

Practice finance

Since the introduction of the NHS in 1948, general practice has grown from a total annual turnover of £5000 per GP to over £350 000 per GP in a funded practice. This means that a group of five GPs in a GP-funded practice will have an annual turnover of £1.75 million.

The **1990 Contract** and the **1991 NHS and Community Care Act** have had major effects on principles and objectives and on financial details.

Objectives

- better value for money through efficiency and market economy policies
- better services and quality of care for patients through built-in checks and audits
- more emphasis on prevention of disease and health promotion.

Details

Achievement of objectives will be effected through:

- new remuneration inducements
- resource management and indicative budgeting for prescribing
- GP fund-holding practices
- better practice management with promotion of computerization, annual reports, audit and teamwork
- encouragement of continuing medical education through Postgraduate Education Allowances (PGEA)

- continuation of reimbursements for employed staff, rates and rent, employing the cost-rent scheme.

New items of service payments

In addition to established principles of annual capitation fees and basic practice allowances, payments have been introduced for a range of new items:

- screening and medical check-ups for new patients, three year non-attenders and over 75s
- child surveillance
- meeting targets for childhood immunization and cervical cytology
- health promotion clinics
- minor surgery
- deprivation (area) allowances
- fees for student attachments.

In addition there are now improved fees for night visits, family planning, maternity services and trainees (*see* page 82).

Costs of NHS General Medical Services

General Medical Services account for over 20% of the total annual expenditure of the NHS. These comprise:

- GPs' medical services   8%
- prescribing by GPs   12%
- FHSA administration   2%
                           _____
                             22%

Figure 13.1: Distribution of General Medical Services costs

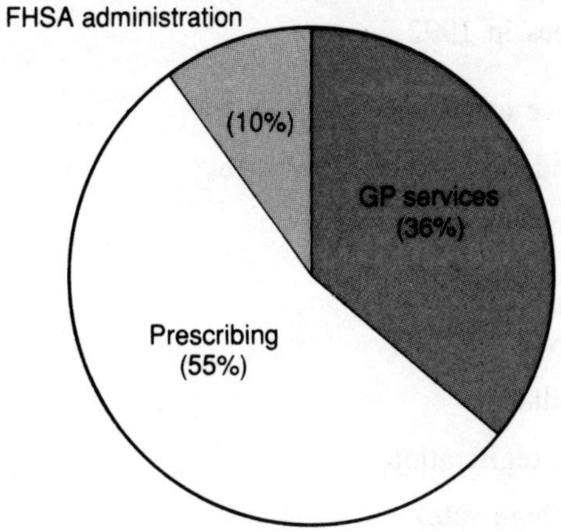

FHSA administration

In 1991–2 this will total around £7.7 billion.

GP income and expenditure

The recommended *income* of a GP for 1991, by the Doctors and Dentists Pay Review Board, was:

Gross	£55 485
Net	£38 465 (less £490 correction).

The recommended *expenditure* of £18 000 per GP was apportioned (%) as follows:

salaries and wages	45
medical supplies	16
premises	13
car travel	7
net capital allowance	4
others	15

(The estimated average whole-time annual salary of an employed staff member in 1991 was £10 000.)

Fees per GP

The rates of fees in 1992 were (£):

- basic practice allowance   6384.00
- seniority and deprivation allowances   flexible
- standard capitation fees
  under 65 year olds   13.85
  65–74 year olds   18.20
  75 and over   35.15
- child surveillance   10.00
- new patient registration   6.10
- night visit (high rate)   45.00
- target meeting for childhood immunization (higher)   1800.00
- target meeting for pre-school immunization (higher)   600.00
- target meeting for cervical cytology (higher)   2280.00
- other vaccination-immunization (fee B)   4.85
- health promotion clinic   45.00
- maternity services (complete)   159.00
- ordinary contraceptive fee   12.75
- family planning (IUCD)   42.75
- minor surgery (per quarter)   100.00
- PGEA (annual)   2025.00
- training   4400.00

In addition, GPs are reimbursed in part for employed staff, rent (cost-rent) and rates.

Fund-holding practices

Under the 1991 NHS and Community Care Act practices with over 9000 (now down to 7000) patients may apply to become 'fund holding'. Such practices are allocated monies to spend on hospital services for their patients. About one in 10 NHS practices is now a fund-holding practice.

The aim is for these practices to commission hospital services for their patients within an agreed budget, and to keep any unspent 'profits' at the end of the year to improve practice services.

The Government's objective was to achieve best value-for-money in a market economy by empowering GPs to 'shop around' the hospitals.

A fund-holding practice has to show that it:

- is able to manage the budget

- has staff to operate the budget

- is computerized to deal with increased management responsibility.

It was hoped that the scheme would result in:

- a wider choice for referral of patients

- an improvement in quality of hospital and GP services

- GPs gaining more control over provision of services

- GPs reducing referrals to hospitals for consultation and investigation by undertaking more in their own practices

- a review of attendances and re-attendances at hospital out-patient departments, and subsequent reduction of these

- promotion of better practice management.

Professor Glennerster has reported some early successes for fund-holding practices in *A foothold for fund holding* (1992).

The GP fund

The fund includes:

- direct clinical referrals for hospital out-patient and some in-patient services and investigations

- domiciliary visits

- direct referrals for physiotherapy, speech therapy, audiology or occupational therapy

- referrals for specific mammography and cervical smears.

It does *not* include:

- acute emergencies
- attendances at hospital accident-emergency services
- self-referrals to hospital
- sexually transmitted diseases
- maternity services
- hearing aids
- neonatal care
- dietetics
- orthoptics
- day care
- child guidance
- chemotherapy and radiotherapy
- renal dialysis
- termination of pregnancy.

From April 1993 community care will be included.

The fund-holding practices negotiate with providers (hospitals) **block fees** to be paid annually to specified hospitals for treating all patients; or **cost and volume** agreed fees for specific types of cases; or on a **cost per case** basis for each individual case. The practices are expected to demand optimal provisions for minimal waiting times at clinics, for appointments and admissions, and for specified standards of care and service.

The practices must send monthly reports and accounts to their FHSAs and RHAs, and they must have a separate bank account for the fund. Any 'profits' go into a reserve fund to be spent on improving patient services.

Annual budget per GP

A GP with 2000 patients, in a fund-holding practice in 1992, can expect to budget on the following basis:

	£
net salary	40 000
prescribing costs (at £50 per patient)	100 000
other income (insurance fees, hospital and other work)	5000
	165 000
Fund (at £100 per patient)	**200 000**
Total income	£365 000

Summary

- Capitation fees now account for 60% of NHS GPs' remuneration.

- New fees for service items are designed to promote prevention and better quality of care.

- General practice and prescribing by GPs account for over 20% of the NHS budget.

- About one in 10 GPs is now in a fund-holding practice. These aim to negotiate more efficient, effective and economic services with hospitals, and carry an added incentive to GPs of making a 'profit' which can be used for improving services for patients.

- The annual gross salary per GP in 1992 is likely to be £60 000 (£40 000 net).

- The 1992 budget per GP in a fund-holding practice is likely to be £365 000.

- The 1992 expenditure per GP on prescribing is likely to be £100 000.

- A review and analysis of the cost-benefits of the new fund-holding arrangements is mandatory.

14

Legislation since 1990 and its effects

The imposition of the Contract for NHS general practitioners in 1990 and the implementation of the NHS and Community Care Act in 1991 have effected the most revolutionary changes on general practice since the introduction of the NHS in 1948. They emphasized better services for patients, more effective and efficient management and more value for NHS monies.

Contractual obligations

Services for patients. Improved availability and accessibility for patients; information on practice organization and services by leaflets (this permitted advertising by doctors); more competition between GPs and choice for patients by increasing income proportion of capitation fees and making it easier for patients to change doctors; and the executive Family Health Service Authority (FHSA) was empowered to ensure good premises and services for patients.

Health promotion. In keeping with national health policies, incentive targets were introduced for remuneration of GPs. These were for:

- immunization of children and cervical cytology smears for women
- health promotion clinics to be funded for approved subjects
- medical check-ups for new registrants and three year non-attender adults
- annual checks on over 75-year-olds as part of extra capitation fees for this group
- child surveillance by examination at set age periods.

Extension of services. Minor surgical procedures were to remunerated in an attempt to reduce referrals to hospital. Night visits by GPs were to receive higher fees. Deprivation allowances would be extra capitation fees for GPs working in designated areas.

Management. All practices were to send annual reports to their FHSA. Computerization was to be encouraged through grants. Staff salary reimbursements were to continue and for more staff, including managers, practice nurses and other para-medical workers. Audit was to be carried out in all practices in the future.

Education. GPs were to receive an annual Postgraduate Education Allowance (PGEA) to enable them to pay for approved continuing medical education; and there were to be fees for teaching medical students and payments for GP trainees on the vocational training scheme.

Fund holding. The most revolutionary item was to encourage internal NHS marketing. Selected large practices were to be given annual funds (budgets) to purchase certain hospital services, for staff pay and prescribing. Any savings could be used by the practice to improve services and facilities.

Since 1990

Targets

In the first year of 1990−1, targets for immunization and cervical cytology were achieved by over 90% of all practices (*see* Table 14.1).

Table 14.1: NHS practices (%) reaching targets for immunization and cervical cytology

	Immunization	Cervical cytology
Higher target	75%	75%
Lower target	15%	20%
	90%	95%

Health promotion clinics

Most practices have carried out some of these clinics for groups of patients. In 1990−1 £44 million was paid to NHS practices for running the clinics. This means an average of £6000 per practice and it also means that the average number of health promotion clinics per practice was 150 or three per week.

Computerization

It is the policy of the NHS to promote computerization in general practice and there have been various forms of financial inducements to achieve this on the assumption that it will lead to better services for patients and saving of money.

The NHS Management Executive commissioned a MORI report on 'GP computing' in 1991.

The Department of Health target was to achieve computerization in 77% of practices. In fact, in 1991, 63% of practices were computerized.

Table 14.2 shows the increases in proportion of computerized practices. The large increase in 1989–90 was in anticipation of the 1990 Contract and in response to subsidization from various quarters.

There were differences between regions. The highest rates of practice computerization were in Oxford (79%), East Anglia (79%), Wessex (77%) and South Western (74%). The lowest rates were in the London (Thames) regions (53–55%). 21% of these practices had Modem links with other computer systems.

Table 14.2: Computerized NHS practices (%)

Year	% NHS practices computerized
1987	10
1988	19
1989	28
1990	47
1991	63
1992 (e)	73
1995 (e)	89

(e = estimate)
Source: NHS Management Executive, MORI Survey 1991

As may be expected, the rate of computerization increased with the size of the practice (by partners) and with fund holding (*see* Table 14.3).

The main users of computer systems were receptionists (93%), GPs (85%) and practice nurses (71%). Practice managers (34%), secretaries (13%) and health visitors (14%) were less frequent users.

Table 14.3: Computerized NHS practices by size and fund holding

Practice size (partners)	% practices computerized
× 1 (single handed)	44
× 2	56
× 3	73
× 4	84
× 5	91
× 6	95
Fund holding	96
Non-fund holding	63
All practices	63

The computers were primarily used for basic non-clinical administration and organization of the practices. Six out of 10 GPs with computers use them during consultations.

Table 14.4: Computer usage rates for clinical and non-clinical functions

Non-clinical	
Patient registration	97%
Repeat prescribing	91%
Call and recall of patients	87%
Appointments	20%
Accounting	17%
Clinical	
Full clinical records	26%
Entry of some clinical data	56%
Annual reports	68%
Audit	59%
Referral letters	34%
Research	27%

The average cost (1990–1) of purchasing of computers was over £10 000 per practice (range £5500–£22 000) and for maintenance almost £1500 (range £552–£3000). Fund-holders spent on average almost £22 000 for their systems, most of which was reimbursed.

Fund holding

Fund holding was the most fiercely debated part of the 1991 NHS and Community Care Act. It was the most radical attempt to move away from a total public NHS monopoly towards a market philosophy: GP practices were to have annual budgets to use, for purchasing a range of hospital services including out-patient consultations, investigations, admissions and certain ancillary services; for the practice prescribing costs; and for paying their staff.

GPs had to become aware of the true costs of medical services. The scheme required enormous amounts of time in preparation, negotiation (with hospitals) and execution. As an experiment, with the first wave of practices, it must be recognized as a remarkably successful achievement, which is a credit to the flexibility and professionalism of the practice teams involved.

The first wave (1990−1) of fund-holding practices all had over 9000 patients, most with five or more partners. They comprised 300 practices with 1700 GPs providing services for some 3 to 3.5 million people.

The second wave (1991−2) contains another 300 practices with some 1500 GPs. This means that in 1992 there are 600 fund-holding practices with 3200 GPs providing services for over six million people or over 10% of UK population.

There is no comprehensive analytical information yet on the results of fund holding, but it appears that the majority of practices like the new system and most have 'profited'.

Audit

Audit was an important theme in the 1990 Contract and the 1991 NHS and Community Care Act. All practices are expected to engage in audit from 1992.

To promote this, each FHSA has been directed to set up a MAAG (Medical Audit Advisory Group) to assist practices. Each MAAG is funded through the FHSA and includes 12 members drawn from local GPs, consultants, an academic, public health physician and medical educator.

Although there are regular published reports on audits from general practice from individuals, there have been no audits published by MAAGs yet and it will be important to make a cost-benefit evaluation of such a nationwide exercise.

Comment

The national economic and political climate in which the 1990 Contract and the 1991 NHS and Community Care Act were introduced was not conducive to an easy birth and neonatal period. There was considerable anger, antipathy and resistance from the medical profession and much anxiety from the public because of fears that the NHS was to be privatized. This was occurring at the time of the parliamentary election in April, 1992. It is all the more remarkable that the 1990 Contract has worked so well.

The numbers of entrants into the GP vocational training programme have gone down, possibly because of adverse publicity and uncertainty about the Contract and the 1991 NHS and Community Care Act. In 1989 there were 2239 trainees in general practice, in 1990 there were 2040 and in 1991 under 2000. As noted in Chapter 5, the replacement number necessary to maintain GP levels is only 1500 so that the reduction to 1900 is not critical; the numbers are likely to increase, simply because there are few other job opportunities in the NHS and little hope for jobs overseas.

15

Future needs

No organization can function efficiently, effectively and economically without access to up-to-date facts and information. Therefore, each part of the NHS must have its own data on which to plan, work, review, change and improve. In addition, there needs to be close correlation and exchange of data between levels.

The data collected must be accurate and reliable, meaningful and practical, applicable and easily collectable. Once collected, the information needs to be reviewed, analysed, discussed and put to good use.

In the NHS, three levels of data collection are evident:

- national

- regional and district

- community and general practice.

National data

National planning for health and provision of medical care must draw on comprehensive macro information. This should include the following.

Demographic data

- population size and distribution

- age and sex – particularly proportions of young people (under 15-year-olds) and the elderly (over 65-year-olds)

- population trends – including birth, fertility and death rates.

Health indices

- life expectancy
- infant mortality
- maternal mortality
- death rates and causes
- preventable deaths
- morbidity
- smoking rates
- rates of and morbidity caused by poverty/deprivation.

Economics

- cost of health care (expressed as % of annual GDP and per capita expenditure)
- sources of funding for health
- distribution of costs amongst hospitals, general practice, and the community.

Resources

- medical, nursing and other manpower
- medical students and new graduates
- distribution of doctors in hospitals and general practice
- unemployment among doctors
- hospital beds and facilities
- community services.

Quality of care

- satisfaction and complaints
- outcomes of care
- utilization rates
- disability rates.

Region and district data

Health authorities at this level are responsible for specialist services, chiefly in hospitals, but also in community care.

There must be data on:

- resources and how they are utilized
- costs, expenditure and cost-benefit ratios
- alternative methods of care and utilization
- quality, standards and outcomes.

Data on the interface between hospital and general practice is of special importance since it is GPs who refer patients to hospitals.

General practice data

Each practice should develop a basic set of data.

This should be primarily for the purposes of planning and organizing the work of the practice in the most effective, efficient and economic ways. It should also serve as material for annual reports to the FHSA and for collaboration with hospital and community services.

Ideally, a nationally agreed set of basic data should be produced and adapted to use in all practices. This should include:

- practice population by age and sex
- staff − numbers and workloads
- work − volume, nature and outcomes
- income, costs, expenditure and profits
- specific items − hospital utilization, prescribing, premises and equipment.

Uses of practice data

Data may be compiled in the following areas as an aid to future planning and improvements.

Staff. Who can do what best? Teamwork, sharing and delegation are important themes.

Work. We need to know how much work we do; how long it takes; its content; and its uses, effects and value. It may be that changes should be made.

Morbidity. We need to know the nature and content of our work and to be aware of its clinical implications; that is to know what are the common conditions, their likely course and outcome, and the most effective ways of managing them. A disease register makes it possible to examine and reconsider our habits of management, and to implement management protocols.

Specific management. As an extension of the disease register, it is useful to keep studies of presentations, diagnoses, treatment (with drugs or other means) and outcomes of defined conditions, and to include costs and medical benefits.

Relations with other services. Referrals for investigations, for out-patient consultation and hospital admissions should be recorded and analysed, as should uses of community and allied services.

Future trends

The NHS, including general practice, has been shaken in the past few years by revolutionary changes towards a new ethos of a 'value for money' market economy.

General practices, pharmacies, community and hopsital services have been forced to plan and re-organize on a data-oriented basis.

New technologies in data collection, storage and analysis have made more things possible.

These trends will continue and health professionals will have to become more familiar and more expert in dealing with statistical information.

References

Much of the data for this book has come from a few sources to which appreciative acknowledgement is made. Additional data has been derived from records from my own practice in Kent.

Association of the British Pharmaceutical Industry (1992) *Pharma facts and figures*. London.

Cancer Research Campaign Reports (1991) London.

Department of Health (1988–91) *Statistics for general medical practitioners for England and Wales*. Statistical bulletins. HMSO, London.

Department of Health (1990–1) *Health and personal social services statistics for England*. HMSO, London.

Department of Health (1991) *General medical practitioners' workload survey 1989–90*. HMSO, London.

Fleming DM (1989) Consulting rates for general practitioners in England. *Journal of the Royal College of General Practitioners*, **39**, 68–72.

Fry J & Sandler G (1988) Domiciliary consultations: some facts and questions. *British Medical Journal*, **297**, 337–9.

General Household Surveys (1989) HMSO, London.

Joint Committee for Postgraduate Training for General Practitioners (1991) Annual report. London.

Kohn R & White KL (1976) *Health Care*. Oxford University Press, Oxford.

Morbidity statistics from general practice (1986) 3rd national study 1981–2. HMSO, London.

Office of Health Economics (1989) *Compendium of health statistics*, 7th edition. OHE, London.

Organization for Economic Co-operation and Development. Reports quoted by OHE.

Parkhouse J (1991) *Doctors' careers*. Routledge, London.

Royal College of General Practitioners (1983) *Present state and future needs*, 6th edition, out of print.

Royal College of General Practitioners (1992) European study of referrals from primary to secondary care. *Occasional Paper 56*.

Social Trends (1989/91), 19th and 21st editions. HMSO, London.

Index